Acupuncture-Moxibustion Therapy

Written   by   Zhang Dengbu
                      Du Guangzhong
Tranlated by   Lu Yubin
                      Lu Yanwei

Shandong Science and Technology Press

First Edition 1996
ISBN 7—5331—1851—0

Acupuncture-Moxibustion Therapy

Written by   Zhang Dengbu

                 Du Guangzhong

Translated by   Lu Yubin

                 Lu Yanwei

Editor in charge Li Yu

Published by Shandong Science and Technology Press
16 Yuhan Road, Jinan, China 250002
Printed by Shandong Binzhou Xinhua Printing House
Distributed by China International Book Trading Corporation
35 Chegongzhuang Xilu, Beijing 100044, China
P. O. Box 399, Beijing, China
Printed in the People's Republic of China

Preface

Acupuncture-Moxibustion Therapy is one volume of *The Series of Traditional Chinese Medicine for Foreign Readers*.

As an important component part of traditional Chinese Medicine, acupuncture-moxibustion has done great contribution to the health of the Chinese nation, and it is now being more and more widely accepted in other countries. However, as acupuncture-moxibustion originates from traditional Chinese culture which is very different from the Western culture, foreign learners often find it very difficult to learn acupuncture-moxibustion well. In order to help foreign acupuncturists especially the acupuncture-moxibustion beginners to study this science well, we compiled this book with its emphasis placed on the introduction of the basic knowledge, basic skills and clinical applications of the acupuncture-moxibustion.

This book consists of eight parts. Each part deals with a special topic concerning acupuncture-moxibustion. Apart from the general knowledge of acpuncture-moxibustion such as the meridians, commonly used acupoints and treatment of diseases with acupuncture-moxibustion, we have also introduced such topic as How to Study Acupuncture-Moxibustion, Auriculo-acupuncture, ELectro-acupuncture and acupuncture anesthesia, with an view to providing the readers with a relatively comprehensive acupuncture-moxibustion knowledge.

This book can work as a textbook for foreign TCM beginners or as a reference for foreign acupuncturists.

Compilers
June, 1996

Contents

A General Introduction to Acupuncture-Moxibustion and Its International Spread and Exchange

An Introduction to Acupuncture-Moxibustion

Acupuncture-moxibustion is a clinical subject dealing with prevention and treatment of diseases with acupuncture-moxibustion under the guidance of theories of traditional Chinese medicine (TCM). As an important part of traditional Chinese medicine and pharmacology, it involves the study of the meridians, acupoints, method of acupuncture-moxibustion, anaesthesia with acupuncture-moxibustion, clinical treatment of diseases with acupuncture-moxibustion and the machanism of the acupuncture-moxibustion.

1. Being an important part of traditional Chinese medicine

Traditional Chinese medicine, a system of knowledge about the

1

life activities and pathologic process of human body as well as prevention, diagnosis and treatment of diseases and the health preservation, comes from summation of the experience of the Chinese people in their long struggle against diseases in the past several thousands years. It contains three parts: the basic medicine, the clinical medicine and the Chinese pharmacology. Of these three parts, the clinical medicine can be divided into such branches as formulas of Chinese drugs, acupuncture-moxibustion, Tuina therapy, Qigong therapy, scrapping therapy, cutting therapy, etc., and acupuncture-moxibustion, thus, serves as a branch of the clinical medicine.

The basic theory of TCM is the theoretical basis for studying and mastering the theories and skills in different clinical branches of traditional Chinese medicine. As an important part of traditional Chinese medicine, acupuncture-moxibustion, naturally, take the basic theory of TCM as its guidance and the meridian theory as its basis, and are conducted in accordance with the syndromes identified through the four diagnostic methods (inquiring, observing, auscultation, palpation) and the eight principles of diagnosis, in order to achieve satisfactory therapeutic effects.

In its long historic development, acupuncture-moxibustion has envoled into a clinical branch of traditional Chinese medicine with rich academic contents and great practical value as a result of the gradual accumulation of the clinical experience and the gradual enrichment of the theory. The academic achievements of acupuncture-moxibustion in the ancient China can be generalized as follows: ① Discovered the meridians communicating with each parts of the human body and established the meridian theory; ② Discovered 361 points of meridians and a great number of extra points, and ascertained the locations and indications of the points; ③ Invented plentiful methods of acupuncture-moxibustion and mastered the indications of acupuncture-moxibustion; ④ Summarized the practical experience in treating different diseases with acupuncture-moxibustion and determined the therapeutic principles such as using the channels in accordance with the syndromes identified, using the points in accordance with channels and administration of different methods in accordance with the syndromes. Thus, the above achievements and the basic theory of TCM, the diagnostic methods and the therapeutic method of TCM, consist of the complete academic system of acupuncture-moxibustion.

2. Acupuncture-moxibustion and acupuncture-moxibustion therapy

Acupuncture-moxibustion is a great contribution of the Chinese nation to the world culture in the field of nature science. People have become more and more familar with it due to its wide spreading. However, the usually mentioned acupuncture-moxibustion has two different meanings. In a broad sense, it indicates acupuncture-moxibustion as a complete academic subject, while in a narrow sense, it means the acupuncture-moxibustion therapy, which is only a part of the subject of acupuncture-moxibustion.

Acupuncture-moxibustion therapy includes the needling therapy, the moxibustion therapy and the special therapies for acupoints developed in the later generations. Although these therapies are applied with different techniques and methods, they are all based on the same theory, or, the basic theory of traditional Chinese medicine or the meridian and acupoints theory which is a part of the basic theory. As for the acupuncture-moxibustion today, the acupuncture-moxibustion therapy includes both the medical and the health preserving techniques with needling or moxibusting as their basic forms despite whether they are conducted at the points or not, and those which are conducted on the points despite whether they are carried out by needling or moxibusting.

3. Clinical application and characteristics of acupuncture-moxibustion

The clinical application of acupuncture-moxibustion mainly includes four aspects which are as follows.

(1) Used to treat diseases and help patient to rehabilitate: Many diseases of different clinical branches, including many functional diseases, infectious diseases and some organic diseases, can be treated with acupuncture-moxibustion. In 1980, World Health Organization suggested that 43 kinds of diseases should be treated with acupunc-

ture-moxibustion in various countries. According to incomplete statistics, acupuncture-moxibustion is being applied to treat more than 300 kinds of diseases of which 100 kinds of diseases or more are very sensitive to the acupuncture-moxibustion treatment, especially various kinds of pains, sensory disturbance, motor impairment and the diseases marked by functional disturbance.

(2) Used to prevent disease and preserve health: Ever since the ancient times, acupuncture-moxibustion has been used to prevent disease and preserve health, with a view to strengthen the constitution and prevent occurrence of diseases. Modern experimental studies also proved that it was capable to increase the immunity of the human body, etc.

(3) Used to induce anaesthesia: Up to today, acupuncture anaesthesia has been adopted in more than 100 kinds of surgical operations. Practice proves that it has the advantages of being safety and effective, bringing about no side and toxic effects or allergic response, exerting less influence on the physiological process, giving quick recovering after operation, and being easy to be performed. Clinically it is commonly used in such operations as thyroidectomy and pulmonary lobeectomy.

(4) Diagnosing disease by means of meridians and acupoints: Examination of such pathological response as pain, numbness or hard nodules occurring in the meridians or acupoints on palpation or determination of the voltage and temperature of the meridians and acupoints can both help to identify the diseased channel, location of disease and the nature of a disease (being deficient or excessive). Besides, needling on related acupoints on a X-ray examination can enhance the accuracy of the X-ray examination.

To summarize, acupuncture-moxibustion has broad indications. However, this doesn't mean that all the diseases can be cured by acupuncture or moxibustion, just like any other therapeutic methods. So, whether acupuncture-moxibustion is adopted or not should be determined based on the practical conditions.

It is just because the acupuncture-moxibustion has the advantage of having broad indications, being highly effective, easy to be conducted, economic and safety, and bringing about no side or toxic effects that they have been widely used and accepted by patients.

4. Origin and development of acupuncture-moxibustion

The acupuncture-moxibustion originates in China. According to the textual research on the literature of the remote antiquity and the unearthed artifacts, acupuncture-moxibustion therapy had been adopted in the Middle and the New Stone Ages which was about 10000—4000 years ago, and its origin can be dated back to the Old Stone Age. At that time, *Bian Shi* (a stone with a sharp adge), bone needle and bamboo needle were used in acupuncture treatment. Afterwards, such needling tools as bronze needle, iron needle, gold needle and silver needle were invented gradually with the development of the casting techniques and the application of the metal tools. Today, stainless steel needle is the most widely adopted needle in the acupuncture treatment. The moxibustion therapy developed gradually after the discovery and application of fire. In the very begining, people in the remote anquity treated diseases through application of hot compression on the diseased area with soil or stone. Afterwards, they adopted the ignited branch of tree or dry grass to treat disease. With the accumulation of experience, they selected the Chinese mugwort leaf as the material for moxibustion treatment.

The acupuncture-moxibustion has experienced a process of gradual development.

During the Spring-Autume and the Warring States Periods (770, BD-221, AD), acupuncture-moxibustion therapy had been widely accepted. The early conditions of acupuncture-moxibustion can be read in the two silk books, *Zu Bi Shi Yi Mai Jiu Jing* (*Moxibustion on the Eleven Channels of Hands and Feet*) and in *Yin Yang Shi Yi Mai Jiu Jing* (*Moxibustion on the Yin-Yang Eleven Channels*), unearthed in the tomb of the Han Dynasty in Changsha City of China in 1973. In the same period, there emerged *Huang Di Nei Jing* (*The Yellow Emperor's Internal Classics*), the earliest classical book on traditional Chinese medicine that can still be read today, which laid the theoretical basis for the further development of acupuncture-moxibustion.

Acupuncture-moxibustion saw its further development from the Qin and Han Dynasties to the Jin Dynasty (221-420 AD.) Zhong Zhongjing, a famous physician of the Han Dynasty, disccussed repeatedly the acupuncture methods and management of errorneous treatment with acupuncture, as well as the combined use of acupuncture and Chinese decoction in treatment of disease in his book *Shang Han Za Bing Lun* (*Treatise On Febrile and Miscellaneous Diseases*). *Zhen Jiu Jia Yi Jing* (*A-B Classic of Acupuncture-Moxibustion*), written by Huangfu Mi in the Jin Dynasty, is the earliest monograph on acupuncture-moxibuston existing today. It made the second great summarization on the acupuncture-moxibustion after *Huang Di Nei Jing* (*The Yellow Emperor's Internal Classic*) and exerted great and remote influence on the development of acupuncture-moxibustion in the later ages.

The period from Sui and Tang Dynasties to the Song and Yuan Dynasties is a period in which the economy of the Chinese society sees its development and prosperity. It is also a period in which the acupuncture-moxibustion makes great progress. Sun Simiao of the Tang Dynasty was the first person suggesting Ah Shi points and he painted the first colourful charts of meridians and acupoints *Ming Tang San Ren Tu*, (*Three Persons' Charts of Mingtang*) which had been lost. In the Sui and Tang Dynasties, a branch specific to acupuncture-moxibustion with professional staffs was set up in the Institute of Loyer Doctors which was in charge of medical education. Wang Weiyi of the North Song Dynasty designed and manufactured two bronze figures of acupuncture-moxibustion, which were considered to be the well-designed figures for medical education in the ancient times as well as an important invention of imaging education in the ancient times. Hua Shou in the Yuan Dynasty believed that the Du and Ren Channels should share the same position with the twleve regular channels and advocated the theory of the fourteen channels. He Ruoyu and Dou Hanqing, two famous acupuncturists in the Jin and Yuan Dynasties, put a high value on selection of points in accordance with different times and the cyclical flow of Qi and Blood in the channels. All these gave an impetus to the development of acupuncture-moxibustion.

The Ming Dynasty (1368-1644 AD.) is the most prosperous period in the development of acupuncture-moxibustion. During this period, many famous acupunturists and monographes on acupuncture-moxibustion emerged. *Zhen Jiu Da Cheng (A Great Compendum of Acupuncture-Moxibustion)* written by Yang Jizhou, which is a summarization of the achievements in acupuncture-moxibustion before the Ming Dynasty, is regared as a new milestone in the development of acupuncture-moxibustion.

During the Qing Dynasty and the Republic of China period (1644-1949 AD.), acupuncture-moxibustion gradually fell into its low ebb as the rulers adopted the polices restricting acupuncture-moxibustion.

After the founding of the people's Republic of China (1949-), acupuncture-moxibustion has seen its rapid development again with the polices on traditional Chinese medicine being practically carried out. It is widely spread all over the country, and, on the basis of inheriting and exploring the ancient acpuncture-moxibustion thoughts, researches by means of modern science and technology are carried out. Great achievements have been obtained in the teaching, clinical treatment and scientific research of acupuncture-moxibustion along with the establishment of universities of traditional Chinese medicine, acupuncture-moxibustion colleges as well as the special researching institutes in the new China. As a result, acupuncture-moxibustion is seeing its upsurge again.

5. The broad prospect of acupuncture-moxibustion

Acupuncture-moxibustion is being deeply explored with advanced scientific and technological techniques actively, so they are deppened in both theory and practice and division of the acupuncture-moxibustion science is becoming more scientific and precise. All the achievements gained in the studies of meridian phenomena, properties of acupoints, relation between visceral organs and the acupoints, the essence of meridians, the histomorphological features of acupoints, the physcial features of acupoints, the biophysical rules of channels and acupoints, the mechanism of holographic structure of the meridians as well as various kinds of hypothesis on the essence of meridians, show that acupuncture-moxibustion has grown to be a new subject including the related contents of both the ancient and the modern, both in China and in foreign countries on a scientific basis.

With the coming of the system and information times, the development of the natural therapy and the rehabilitating cause, the enhancement of the therapeutic effects of acupuncture, as well as the constant emerging of the scientific achievements in the study of acupuncture-moxibustion, the world will need acupuncture-moxibustion more and more, thus, acupuncture-moxibustion has a bright future.

International Spread and Exchange of Acupuncture-Moxibustion

As early as in the ancient times, acupuncture-moxibustion had been introduced from China to other countries, especially the neighbours of China. As an important content of medical exchanges between China and other countries, it has made some contributions to the health of the peopel of all the world.

1. A history of international spread and exchange of acupuncture-moxibustion

As early as in 500 AD. , *Zhou Hou Jiu Cu Fang* (*Prescriptions for Emergency*), a comprehensive book of medicine containing acupuncture-moxibustion, had been introduced into Japan. In 552, China sent the Mikado of Qingming a set of *Zhen Jing* (*Acupuncture-Moxibustion Classis*). Ten years later, Zhi Cong from Wu State of China went to Japan taking *Ming Tang Tu* (*A Charts of Acupuncture-Moxibustion*)and *Zhen Jiu Jia Yi Jing* (*An A-B Classic of Acupuncture-Moxibustion*) with him. In 701, Department of Acupuncture-moxibustion began to be set up in the institutes of medical education. In 808, based on the books *Su Wen* (*The Plain Questions*), *Huang Di Zhen Jing* (*Huang Di's Classic of Acupuncture*), *Zhen Jiu Jia Yi Jing* (*An A-B Classic of Acupunture and Moxibustion*) and *Xiao Pin Fang* (*Minute Prescriptions*), the Japanese doctors compiled the book *Da Tong Lei Ju Fang* (*Prescriptions Assigned In Accordance with Syndromes*) which contained one handred volumes. Acupuncture-moxibustion experienced a rapid development in Japan from Nala to Heian periods with some original creation. In Edo period, acupuncture-moxibustion had reached a higher level in Japan, and plenty of acupuncture books were published. After the Meiji Reformation in Japan, acupuncture was repelled until the 60's of the 19th century. In 1867, a famous Japanese doctor began to do experimental study on the acupuncture-moxibustion for the first time, holding that the mechansim of treating disease with acupuncture-moxibustion was related to the nervous system. In 1907, an article about the influence of acupuncture on some physiological phenomena was published. Since then, more and more people have been involved in the experimental study of acupuncture-moxibustion.

In 541, China began to send doctors to Korea and consequently acupuncture-moxibustion was introduced to Korea. In 692, doctor of acupuncture began to teach students in a special department set up by the Xinluo dynasty, with *Zhen Jing* (*Acupuncture Classic*) and *Ming Tang Tu* (*A Charts of Acupuncture-Moxibustion*) as the textbooks. By the Song and Yuan Dynasties of China, many acupuncture-moxibustion books such as *Zhen Jiu Zi Sheng Jing* (*A Classic of Saving Life with Acupuncture-Moxibustion*) and *Shi Si Jing Fa Hui* (*An Elucidation of the Fourteen Channels*) had been transmitted to Korea successively. In the same time, the Korean also compiled such books with special thoughts of Korean people as *Xiang Yao Ji Cheng* (*A Collection of Countryside Medicine*), *Yi Fang Lei Ju* (*A Compendum of Assigned Medical Formulas*) and *Zhen Jiu Ze Ri Bian Ji* (*A Collection of Acupuncture on A Chosen Day*) all of which contained the acupuncture-moxibustion. Since the acupuncture-moxibustion was introduced into Japan and Korea, they have been a part of their traditional medicine up to today.

With the cutural exchange between China and foreign countries, acupunture and moxibustion were also transmitted to South-East countries as well as other countries and regions of Asia such as India. In 14th century, Zhou Geng, an acupunturist from China once went to Viet Nam to treat diseases for its high officers and was praised to be a holy doctor there.

In the European and American countries, there was rarely records on acupunture-moxibustion before 17th century. With the increase of cultural exchanges between China and foreign countries, acupunture-moxibustion were gradually understood and partly adopted in these countries. In 1658, Dane. Jacob. Bondt introduced acupuncture therapy; in 1676, Buschof, H. , etc. , introduced moxibustion therapy; and in 1683, Rhijne, W. made a detailed discussion on acupuncture therapy in his book *On Acupunture Therapy*. In the 18th century and the first half of the 19th century, acupuncture-moxibustion was more widely spread and introduced. About 47 kinds of acupunture books were published in such European and American countries as the France, the Great Britain, Germany, the United States, Italia and Russia. From the middle age of the 19th century to the middle age of the 20th century, Soulie · de · Morant, G. and Dela · Fuye from France, Bertarelli. E. from Italy, Фолворт from Russia, etc. , contributed greatly to the transmission of acupuncture-moxibustion in the European and American countries.

2. Present situation of international spread and exchange of acupuncture-moxibustion

With the wide international transmission and exchange of acupuncture-moxibustion, more than 120 countries and regions have possessed their own acupuncture doctors who are treating diseases with acupuncture-moxibustion, academic organizations of acupuncture-moxibustion has been set up in about 55 countries, and more than ten international organization of acupuncture-moxibustion has been carried out their activities. So the tendency of internationzation of acupuncture-moxibustion is increasing.

Japan is the representative of the tendency in Asia. At present, there are more than 60,000 acupunturists, more than 30 schools of acupuncture-moxibustion, 2 universities, 20 or more acupuncture associations, more than 10 kinds of acupunture journals such as The Journal of All Japan Acupunture Association, and about 20 researching institutes of acupuncture-moxibustion in Japan. Japanese have suggested the favorable meridian-inducing therapy and found the papula emerging along the distribution route of channels. In recent years, more and more clinical and experimental reports occurred. In addition to Japan, acupuncture-moxibustion is also being widely spread and adopted in such Asian countries as Korea, India, Sri Lanka, Pakistan, the Philippines, Viet Nam and Singapore.

Acupuncture-moxibustion is most prevalent in France in Europe. Now, there are about 4000 acupuncturists. 10 acupuncture schools, 18 acupuncture associations and researching institutes, and 5 kinds of acupuncture journals in France. In recent years, faculty of acupuncture has been set up in almost all the medical colleges or universities, and the French doctors have advocated the auricular acupuncture therapy of the French style. In Russia, there are about 10000 acupuncturists at present, most of whom are those trained with acupuncture-moxibustion after graduated from colleges of Western medicine. They apply acupuncture-moxibustion in their clinical work and have suggested the "Reflexion Therapy". In addition, acupuncture-mosibustion is also widely adopted in such European countries as Germany, Astria, Italy, Finland, Holland, the Great Britain, Polland and Hungary.

In the America, the United States and Canada also attach great importance to acupuncture-moxibustion. In the past 10 years, about 2.5 millions American have experienced the acupuncture-moxibustion treatment, and about 10000 people are engaged in the clinical or research work of acupuncture in the United States. Besides, there are more than 20 acupuncture associations and six kinds of journals including American Journal of Acupuncture are published in the United States. Acupuncture education also progresses rapidly, especially in California, which posesses 4 acupuncture colleges and more than 10 acupuncture schools, and such new theory as Holographic

Theory of Meridians has been put forward. Besides, acupuncture-moxibustion has also effeciently spread and adopted in such countries as Argentina, Canada and Mexico in the America, Egypt and Nigeria in Africa, and Australia and New Zealand in the Pacific area.

The acupuncture-moxibustion is not only adopted, researched and appreciated, but also developed in more and more countries. Apart from the above mentioned, such therapies as Korea Finger Therapy, Fu'er Electro-acupuncture Therapy, Face Diagnosis and Back-feeding Therapy, Skeleton-Needling Therapy, Colour-Bright Acupuncture Therapy, TEN'S Therapy and SSP Therapy are all the new therapies invented by foreign scholars based on the Chinese acupuncture-moxibustion, which have enriched the academic thoughts of acupuncture-moxibustion. New ideas about the essence of meridians and the experimental studies on the mechanism of acupuncture-moxibustion is almost countless. Such studies as application of acupuncture-moxibustion in the treatment of AIDS in the America and the application of acupuncture in correcting the malaise of the astronauts induced by weightlessness have extended the scope of the acupuncture-moxibusiton study.

In addition, founding of the International Acupuncture Association, the successful opening of the international training course of acupuncture-moxibustion in China and the drawing of the standard normenclature of acupoints will be a great impetus to the wide spread and exchanges of acupuncture-moxibustion throughout the world, pushing the invention and development of acupuncture-moxibustion science forwards. We believe that acupuncture will finally become an inseparable part of the World medicine.

How to Learn Acupuncture-Moxibustion

*W*ith the wide spread and exchange of acupuncture-moxibustion throughout the world, the science of acupuncture-moxibustion is growing to be an organic part of the world medicine. Peoples in most countries hope that they have the chance to study acupuncture-moxibustion systematically. However, as the academic system of acupuncture-moxibustion today comes from summarization of the experience of the ancient Chinese people in their long struggle against diseases and serves as a product of the ancient Chinese scientific thoughts, it has different ways of thinking compared with the Western medicine in the understanding of the human body and the complicated disease. Therefore, it is necessary for foreigners to study acupuncture-moxibustion with a new mind and a multiple dimension thoughts, in order to study and master the acupuncture-moxibustion at a high level.

13

Method of Learning
Acupuncture-Moxibustion

1. Paying more attentions to basic theory of traditional Chinese medicine

Being an inseparable part of traditional Chinese medicine, acupuncture-moxibustion takes the basic theory of TCM as its guidance and the meridian theory as its basis. So, one must learn and master the basic theory of traditional Chinese medicine well in order to study acupuncture-moxibustion, otherwise, he or she will fail to diagnose diseases, determine the therapeutic methods in accordance with the syndromes, select points and manipulate the needles correctly, and thus good therapeutic effects cannot be expected. Many foreign friends are not aware that they have lowered the scientific position of acupuncture-moxibustion to be so low as the simple acupuncture-moxibustion therapy as a result of their neglecting the study of the basic theory of traditional Chinese medicine, and just because of this, they fail to grasp the core of the academic system of acupuncture-moxibustion. Therefore, it is very important to learn the basic theory of traditional Chinese medicine well.

2. Strengthening the training of the basic skills of acupuncture-moxibustion

Acupuncture-moxibustion is a subject of medicine with complete theory and strong practical or technical nature. So, acupuncturist must master the basic skills for acupuncture-moxibustion treatment well. Better therapeutic effects cannot be achieved in the case of failure to manipulate the needle nimbly and insert the needle smoothly, failure to induce the feeling of gaining Qi after insertion or failure to exert such manipulations as reinforcing and reducing, and in the case of occurrence of severe pain after inserting. Therefore, it is an immportant link in the study of acupuncture-moxibustion to strengthen the training of the basic skills for acupuncture-moxibustion treatment.

3. Having a good knowledge of the names and meanings of the acupoints

Names of acupoints are very important component parts of the acupuncture terms. They have not only meanings of medicine, but also have the meanings of the brilliant ancient Chinese culture. As a whole, the acupoints are named after their locations and actions, the achievements of scientific research in the ancient times and the theories of Chinese medicine. For example, Wangu (GB 12) located near the wrist and Rugen (ST 18) located below the breasts, are named after the names of the anatomical structure where the points are located or the features of the place the points are located; Guangming (GB 37), which means brightness, can be used to treat eye disease, and Shuifen (RN9), which can be used to treat ascite or edema, is named after its indication, etc.

Attentions for Studying
Acupuncture-Moxibustion

Acupuncture-moxibustion is a medical skill with a strong clinical feature. Apart from mastering the basic knowledge of acupuncture-moxibustion such as the meridians and acupoints, one should pay attentions more in his/her study to the clinical practice more and should be persistent in doing the clinical practice.

1. Practising more in the clinic

Acupuncture-moxibustion is a clinical branch of traditional Chinese medicine. So, one must combine what he has learnt with his clinical practice. Only through careful observation and comprehensive analysis of diseases in the clinic under the guidance of the basic theories, can he find the channels involved in identification of syndromes, select the points correctly according to the distribution of channels, and apply different therapeutic methods in accordance

15

with the different syndromes. And through the clinical practice, he can constantly enhance his level of both the clinical treatment and the basic theory.

2. Step by step in the study with a steady spirit

There are a lots of basic knowledge, basic concepts and basic skills to be learnt in the academic system of acupuncture-moxibustion which contains the essentials, manipulations and clinical applications of acupuncture-moxibustion. So, it is impossible to learn all these well in a short time and thus one should spend his time constantly on study of acupuncture-moxibustion.

Meridians

*T*he meridian theory is a subject that deals with the distribution, physiological functions, pathological changes of the different channels of the human body as well as their relations with the Zang-Fu organs. It is an important component part of traditional Chinese medicine, and as it has been accomplished early, it has played a leading role in the formation of the theoretical system of traditional Chinese medicine. Since its formation, it has been guiding the clinical practice of the different branches of traditional Chinese medicine, especially the acupuncture-moxibustion.

Meridian is a collective name for both the channels and the collaterals. Channels are the main trunk of the meridians which are mainly distributed vertically; while the collaterals are the branches separating from the channels and functioning to connect with every part of the body like a network. Through the connecting function of the meridians, the interior and the exterior of the human body, the Zang-Fu organs and the limbs are intergrated into an unity.

Components of the Meridian System

The meridian system includes the twelve regular channels, the eight extraordinary channels and the fifteen major collaterals as well as the twelve muscular regions and the twelve cutaneous regions attached to them.

1. The twelve regular channels

The twelve regular channels are the main trunk of the meridian system. They are named after their different Yin-Yang natures, their different pertaining Zang or Fu organs and their different distributing routes. Each of the twelve regular channels pertains to a Zang organ or a Fu organ. The channel distributed in the medial aspect of the limbs belongs to Yin and pertains to the Zang organ, while that distributed in the lateral aspect of the limbs belongs to Yang and pertains to Fu organ. The channels running in the upper limbs are called the hand channels; while those going in the lower limbs, the foot channels. The twelve regular channels are distributed in the medial or the lateral aspects of the upper limbs or the lower limbs, and in each aspect there are three channels. So, one Yin and one Yang evolve into three Yin and three Yang, namely, Taiyin, Shaoyinyin, Jueyin, Yangming, Taiyang and Shaoyang respectively, which are identified according to the vicissitude of Yin Qi or Yang Qi.

The twelve regular channels, due to communication and link of their branches and the collaterals, form six groups of pertaining-connecting relations with the Zang-Fu organs. That is, the Yin channels pertain to Zang organs and connect with the Fu organs; and the Yang channels pertain to Fu organs and connect with the Zang organs. And through the connexions of the hand and the foot channels, the Yin and Yang channels and the interior-exteriorly related channels, the twelve regular channels form a circular system in which Qi and Blood flow through the cnannels one by one endlessly. The cyclical flow of Qi and Blood and the connexion place of the twelve regular channels are as follows:

The Lung Channel of Hand-Taiyin ⇒ at the tip of the middle finger ⇒ The Large Intestine Channel of Hand-Yangming ⇒ beside the nose ⇒ The Stomach Channel of Foot-Yangming ⇒ at the tip of the great toe ⇒ The Spleen Channel of Foot-Taiyin ⇒ in the Heart ⇒

18

The Heart Channel of Hand-Shaoyin ⇒ at the tip of the little finger ⇒ The Small Intestine Channel of Hand-Taiyang ⇒ in the inner cannthus ⇒ The Bladder Channel of Foot-Taiyang ⇒ at the tip of the little toe ⇒ The Kidney Channel of Foot-Shaoyin ⇒ in the chest ⇒ The Pericardium Channel of Hand-Jueyin ⇒ At the tip of the ring finger ⇒ The Triple-Jiao Channel of Hand-Shaoyang ⇒ at the outer canthus ⇒ The Gallbladder Channel of Foot-Shaoyang ⇒ in the great toe ⇒ The liver Channel of Foot-Jueyin ⇒ in the Lung ⇒ the Lung Channel of Hand-Taiyin.

The distributing routes of the twelve regular channels are as follows:

(1) The Lung Channle of Hand-Taiyin: The Lung Channel of Hand-Taiyin originates from the Middle-Jiao, running downward to connect with the large intestine. Winding back, it goes along the lower orifice (the duodenum) and the upper orifice (the cardia) of the stomach, passes through the diaphragm, and enters the lung, its pertaining organ. Then it goes upward to the throat where it runs transversely to the laterosuperior side of the chest. Emerging in the axillary fossa, it runs downward along the anterior border of the medial aspect of the upper arm, passes through the cubital fossa and enters Cunkou (the radial artery at the wrist for pulse palpation). Passing through the thenar eminence, it reaches the tip of the thumb (Shaoshang, LU11)..

The branch proximal to the wrist emerges from Lieque (LU 7) and runs directly to the radial side of the tip of the index finger (Shangyang, LI1) where it links with the Large Intestine Channel of Hand-Yangming.

(2) The Large Intestine Channel of Hand-Yangming: The Large Intestine Channel starts from the tip of the radial side of the index finger (Shangyang, LI1). Passing through the dorsum of hand, it travels along the anterior border of the lateral aspect of the arm to the shoulder. Then it goes in front of the shoulder joint backward to the point below the spinous process of the 7th cervical vertebra (Dazhui, DU 14). From there, it goes forwards, entering the supraclavicular fossa to connect with the lung in the thorax. Descend-

19

ing, it passes through the diaphragm to reach the large intestine, its pertaining organ.

The branch emerging in the supraclavicular fossa goes upward along the side of the neck and the cheek to enter the lower gum. Winding back, it runs around the corners of mouth and crosses the opposite channel at philtrum, ending at the opposite side of the nose (Yingxiang, Li20), where it links with the Stomach Channel of Hand-Yangming.

(3)The Stomach Channel of Foot-Yangming: The Stomach Channel of Foot-Yangming starts from the lateral side of ala nasi (Yingxiang, LI 20). It then ascends along the side of the nose to the bridge of the nose where it goes laterally to enter the inner canthus to meet with the Bladder Channel of Foot-Taiyang. Turning downwards along the lateral side of the nose, it enters the upper gum. Reemerging, it curves around the lips and descends to meet the opposite channel at the mentaolabial groove (Chengjiang, RN 24). Then it goes posterolaterally across the portion of the cheek at Daying (ST 5.) Winding back along the mandible, it ascends in front of the ear and transverses Shangguan (GL 3). Then it follows the anterior hairline and reaches the forehead.

The facial branch emerging in front of Daying (ST 5) runs downwards to Renying (ST 9). From there, it goes along the throat posteriorly to Dazhui (DR 14). Then it winds back and enters the supraclavicular fossa. Descending, it passes through the diaphragm, enters the stomach, its pertaining organ, and connects with the spleen.

The straight portion of the channel arises from the supraclavicular fossa. It runs downwards, passing through the nipple. It then descends by the umbilicus and enters Qichong (ST 30) on the groin.

The branch from the lower orifice of the stomach descends inside the abdomen and joints the previous portion of the channel at Qichong (ST 30). Then it runs downwards along the anterior aspect of the thign, reaching the knee. Descending further, it goes along the anterior border of the lateral aspect of the tibia, passes through the dorsum of foot and enters the lateral side of the tip of the second toe.

The tibial branch arises from Zusanli (ST 36), three cun below the knee, and enters the lateral side of the third toe.

The branch from the dorsum of the foot emerges from Chongyang (ST 42), ending at the medial side of the tip of the greater toe (Yinbai SP 1), where it links with the Spleen Channel of Foot-Taiyin.

(4) The Spleen Channel of Foot-Taiyin: The Spleen Channel of Foot-Taiyin starts from the medial side of the greater toe (Yinbai SP 1). It runs along the medial aspect of the foot at the junction of the red and white skin, and ascends in front of the medial malleolus up to the leg, where it goes along the midline of the medial aspect of the leg. At the point eight cun above the medial malleolus, it crosses and goes in front of the Liver Channel of the Foot-Jueyin. Passing through the anterior medial aspect of the thigh, it enters the abdomen, then the spleen, its pertaining organ and connects with the stomach. From there it ascends, passing through the diaphragm and runing alongside the esophagus. When it reaches the root of the tongue, it spreads over its lower surface.

The branch from the stomach goes upward through the diaphragm, and flows into the heart to link with the Heart Channel of Hand-Shaoying.

(5) The Heart Channel of Hand-Shaoyin: The Heart Channel of Hand-Shaoyin starts from the heart. Emerging, it spreads over the "heart system". Passing through the diaphragm, it goes downward to connect with the small intestine.

The branch emerging from the heart system goes alongside the esophagus upwards to connect with the "eye system".

The straight portion of the channel arises from the heart system, then it goes upwards to the lung, where it turns downwards and emerges from the axilla (Jiquan, HT 1). Going along the posterior border of the medial aspect of the upper arm, it passes through the tip of the elbow and reaches the pisiform region proximal to the palm. Then it follows the medial aspect of the little finger to its tip (Shaochong HT 9) and links with the Small Intestine Channel of Hand-Taiyang.

21

(6) The Small Intestine Channel of Hand-Shaoyang: The Small Intestine Channel of Hand-Shaoyang originates from the ular side of the little finger (Shaoze, SI 1). Going along the posterior border of the dorsum of hand and the lateral aspect of the forearm, it passes through the elbow to the posterior border of the shoulder joint. From there, it runs around the scapula to meet the opposite channel at Dazhui (DU 14). Then it travels forwards to enter the supraclavicular fossa. Inside the body cavities, it connects with the heart, and alongside the esophagus, it passes through the diaphragm to the stomach, where it continues to descend to the small intestine, its pertaining organ.

The branch from the supraclavicular fossa reaches the cheek along the neck, then it ascends to the outer canthus and goes backwards to enter the ear (Tinggong, SI 19).

The branch from the cheek ascends to the infraorbital region and further to the inner canthus (Jingming, BD 1), where it links with the Bladder Channel of Foot-Taiyang.

(7) The Bladder Channel of Foot-Taiyang: The Bladder Channel of Foot-Taoyang starts at the inner canthus (Jingming, BD 1). Ascending to the forehead, it joins its opposite channel at the vertex (Baihui, DU 20).

The branch arising from the vertex goes to the temple.

The straight portion of the channel goes backward and downward to the occipital region to enter and communicate with the brain. Turning back. it descends to the posterior aspect of the neck, meeting its opposit channel at Dazhui (DU 14). Then it bifurcates and travels 1. 5 cun lateral to the medial side of the scapula and the spinal column, reaching the lumbar region, where it enters the body cavity via the paravertebral muscle to connect with the kidney and joint the bladder, its pertaining organ.

The branch arising from the lumbar region descends beside the spinal column. Passing through the gluteal region, it travels downwards to the popliteal fossa along the lateral side of the posterior aspect of the thigh.

The branch originating from the posterior aspect of the neck goes in the medial side of the scapular region. At Fufen (UB 41), it runs downwards 3 cun lateral to the spinal column to the hip joint. Then it goes along the posterior aspect of the thigh to meet the previous branch in the popliteal fossa. Going further downwards, it passes through the gastrocnemius muscle and emerges behind the external malleolus. From there, it runs along the lateral border of the dorsum of foot to terminate at the tip of the lateral side of the little toe (Zhiyin, KI 1), where it links with the Kidney Channel of Foot-Shaoyin.

(8) The Kidney Channel of Foot-Shaoyin: The Kidney Channel of Foot-Shaoyin starts from the inferior aspect of the small toe and runs obliquely to the sole (Yongquan, KI 1). Emerging from the lower aspect of the tubersity of the navicular bone, it runs behind the medial malleolus and enters the heel. Then it ascends along posterior border of the medial side of the leg to the medial side of the popliteal fossa and further upward along the postero-medial aspect of the thign towards the spinal column (Changqiang, DU 1). Passing through the spinal column, it enters the kidney, its pertaining organ, and connects with the bladder.

The straight portion of the channel goes upwards from the kidney. Passing through the liver and the diaphragm, it enters the lung and alongside the throat, reaches the bilateral sides of the root of the tongue.

The branch arising from the lung connects with the heart and flows into the thorax to link with the Pericardium Channel of Hand-Jueyin.

(9) The Pericardium Channel of Hand-Jueyin: The Pericardium Channel of Hand-Jueyin originates from the thorax. Emerging, it communicates with the pericardium, its pertaining organ. Passing through the diaphragm, it connects with the Upper-Jiao, the Middle-Jiao and the Lower-Jiao successively.

The branch arising from the thorax emerges from the costal region 3 cun below anterior axillary fossa (Tianchi, PC 1). It then ascends to the axilla and travels along the midline of the medial aspect of the upper arm to enter the cubital fossa. Passing through the wrist, it enters the center of the palm (Laogong, PC 8) and further goes along the radial side of the middle finger to its tip (Zhong-chong, PC 9).

The branch from the palm goes to the tip of the ring finger along its ulnar side to link with the Triple-Jiao Channel of Hand-Shaoyang.

(10) The Triple-Jiao Channel of Huand-Shaoyang: The Triple-Jiao Channel of Hand-Shaoyang starts from the ulnar side of the tip of the ring finger (Guanchong, SJ 1). Going upwards along the ul-nar side of the ring finger, it reaches the dorsum of the hand. Then it goes upward between the ulna and the radius in the forearm. Passing through the olecranon and along the lateral aspect of the up-per arm, it enters the supraclavicular fossa from the shoulder, spreads over the thorax to connect with the pericardium. Passing through the diaphragm, it communicates with the Upper-Jiao, the Middle-Jiao and the Lower-Jiao successively.

The branch from the thorax goes upwards to emerge in the supra-clavicular fossa. Reaching the shoulder, it meets its opposite chan-nel at Dazhui (DU 14). Then, it ascends on the posterior aspect of the neck where along the posterior region of the ear, it goes up to the temple. Then it curves downwards. Passing through the cheek, it reaches the infraorbital region.

The branch arising from the posterior region of the ear enters the ear and reemerges in front to the ear. Crossing the previous branch in cheek, it terminates at the outer canthus (Tongzliao, GB 1) to link with the Gallbladder Channel of Foot-Shaoyang.

(11) The Gallbladder Channel of Foot-Shaoyang: The Gallblad-der Channel of Foot-Shaoyang originates from the outer canthus (Tongziliao, GB 1), ascends to the corner of the forehead (Hanyan, GB 4), then curves downwards to the retroauricular region (Wan-gu, GB 12). From there, it ascends and curves, passing through the forehead, to the supraorbital region, curves backward and downward to the retroauricular region again (Fengchi, GB 20) and runs along the side of the neck to the shoulder. Then it meets its opposite at Dazhui (DU 14) and runs forward to enter the supra-

clavicular fossa.

The branch from the retroauricular region enters the ear and reemerges in front of the ear, reaching the posterior border of the outer canthus.

The branch arising from the outer canthus runs downwards and meets the branch of the Triple-Jiao Channel of Hand-Shaoyang at Daying (Gb ST 5), then it goes to the infraorbital region. The branch going downward passes through the mandible of the jaw and the neck, meeting the previous channel in the supraclavicular fossa. Then, it enters the body cavity. Passing through the diaphragm, it connects with the liver and reaches the gallbladder, its pertaining organ. From there, it runs inside the hypochondriac region. Coming out from the groin, it runs along the margin of the public hair and transverses to the hip region (Huantiao, GB 30).

The straight portion of the channel runs downward from the supraclavicular fossa, passes in front of the axilla along the lateral aspect of the chest and through the free end of the ribs to the hip region where it meets the previous branch. Then it descends along the lateral aspect of the thigh to the lateral side of the knee. Going further downward along the anterior border of the fibula all the way to its lower end, it emerges from the anterior aspect of the external malleolus and follows the dorsum of the foot to the lateral side of the tip of the 4th toe (Zuqiaoyin, GB 44).

The branch from the dorsum (Zulingqi, GB 41) of the foot goes forwards to the lateral aspect of the big toe, then it turns back, passing through the nail, and terminates at its hairy region, where it links with the Liver Channel of Foot-Jueying.

(12) The Liver Channel of Foot-Jueyin: The Liver Channel of Foot-Jueyin originates from the hairy region of the great toe. Runing upward along the dorsum of the foot, passing through Zhongfeng (LR 4), which is 1 cun in front of the medial malleolus, it ascends to an area 8 cun above the medial malleolus, where it runs across and behind the Spleen Channel of Foot-Taiyin. Then it runs further upwards to the medial aspect of the knee and along the medial aspect of the thigh to enter the public hairy region, where it

curves around the external genitalia and goes up to the lower abdomen. It then runs upward alongside the stomach to reach the liver, its pertaining organ and connect with the gallbladder. From there, it continues to ascend, passing through the diaphragm and branching out from the costal and hypochondriac region. Then it runs upwards along the posterior aspect of the throat, entering the nasopharharynx and connects with the "eye system". Running upwards further, it emerges from the forehead and, goes upward further and meets the Du Channel at the vertex.

The branch from the eye system runs downward into the cheek, and curves around the inner surface of the lips.

The branch arising from the liver, passing through the diaphragm, goes upward to enter the lung, linking with the Lung Channel of Hand-Taiyin.

2. The eight extrordinary channels

The eight extraordinary channels include the Du Channel. the Ren Channel, the Chong Channel, the Dai Channel, the Yinwei Channel, the Yangwei Channel, the Yinqiao Channel and the Yangqiao Channel. Different from the twelve regular channels, they are so-called because they haven't direct pertaining relations with Zang-Fu organs and the interior-exterior relationships among them, and are not so regular in distribution as the twelve regular channels. Most of related points of the eight extraordinary channels are located in the twelve regular channels except for the points of the Du and Ren Channels which are in these two channels. So the Ren and Du Channels and the twelve regular channels are collectively called the fourteen channels.

The eight extraordinary channels are distributed vertically and horizontally among the twelve regular channels, so they have two major functions: ① Communicating with the twelve regular channels and thus strengthening the connections among the twelve regular channels. The Du Channel is related to the six Yang channels, so it can regulate the Qi of all the Yang channels of the body; the Ren Channel is related to the six Yin channels, so it can regulate the Qi of all the Yin channels of the body; the Chong Channel is related to the Du Channel, the Ren Channel, the Stomach Channel of Hand-Yangming and the Kidney Channel of Foot-Shaoyin, so it has the function of storing Qi and Blood from the twelve regular channels; the controlling effect of the Dai Channel can strengthen the connections of the vertically distrbuted channels of foot; the Yinwei Channel and the Yangwei Channel connect with the Yin channels and the Yang channels of the whole body respectively and dominate the exterior and the interior of the human body; and the Yinqiao Channel and the Yangqiao Channel are in charge of movement and stillness of the human body respectively, so they functions together to control the movements of the lower limbs and sleeping and waking. ②Having a regulatory effect on Qi and Blood of the twelve regular channels. When Qi and Blood in the twelve regular channels are exuberant, they flow into the eight extraordinary channels to be stored; while when more Qi and Blood are needed to support the functional activities of the meridians and Zang-Fu organs, Qi and Blood will flow from the extraordinary channels to supply for the activities.

The distributing routes of the eight extraordinary channels are as follows:

(1) The Du Channel: It originates inside the lower abdomen. Running downward, it emerges in the perineum. Then, it runs upward inside the spinal column to Fengfu (DU 16) in the nape, where it enters and connects with the brain. Turning back, it continues to go upward to the vertex. Then, it runs downward along the midline of the forehead. Passing through the root of the nose, it ends at Yinjian (RN 7) in the frenulum of the upper lip.

(2) The Ren Channel: Originating inside the lower abdomen, this channel goes downward and emerges in the perineum. Then it runs upward, enter the public hairy region. Going upward further inside the abdomen, it goes along the anterior midline of the body and passes through such points as Guanyuan (RN 4), reaching the throat. Then it continues to run upward, runs around the lips, passes through the face and ends in the infraorbital region.

(3) The Chong Channel: This channel originates inside the lower

abdomen. Then, it runs downwards and emrges in the perineum. In where the pulsation is felt in the groin, it goes together with the Kidney Channel of Foot-Shaoyin. Running upward, it goes alongsides the umbilicus, reaching the chest and diffusing in the thoracic cavity. Then it goes further upward, passes through the throat, goes around the lips and terminates in the infraorbital region. One of its branches originates from the Kidney together with the major collaterals of the Kidney Channel of Foot-Shaoyin. Then it runs downwards and emerges in the groin, where it runs downward along the medial aspect of the thigh and enters the popliteal fossa. From there, it continues to go deeply downward along the medial side of the tibia in the lower leg, reaching the upper border of the calcaneus behind the tip of the medial malleolus and then the foot. Its branch arises from the channel behind the malleolus, goes forwards obliquely to the dorsum of foot and enters the great toe. Another branch of the channel comes out from the main channel inside the lower abdomen, goes backward to communicate with the Du Channel and travels upwards inside the spinal column.

(4) The Dai Channel: This channel starts from the inferior region of the hypochondrium. Then, it goes downward obliquely to Daimai (GB 26) and goes transversely around the waist. The portion of the channel in the abdomen droops to the lower abdomen.

(5) The Yinqiao Channel: This channel comes out from the Kidney Channel of Foot-Shaoyin at Zhaohai (KI 6) below the malleolus. Then, it goes upward behind the malleolus to the medial aspect of the lower limbs, entering the public region. Then, it further goes upward along the abdomen and chest to enter the supraclavicular fossa. Going upward further, it emerges in front of Renying (ST 9), passes by the nose and terminates at the inner canthus, where it meets with the Yangqiao Channel and the Taiyang channels of both hand and foot.

(6) The Yangqiao Channel: This channel comes out from the Bladder Channel of Foot-Taiyang at Shenmai (UB 62) below the external malleolus. Then, it runs upward behind the external malleolus. Passing through the abdomen and the posterolateral aspect of

the chest, it goes around the corner of the mouth and reaches the inner canthus, where it meets with the Yinqiao Channel and the Taiyang channels of both hand and foot. From there, it continues to go upward, enters the hair and then descends to the retroauricular region and the nape, where it meets with the Gallbladder Channel of Foot-Shaoyang.

(7) The Yinwei Channel: This channel starts at Zhubin (KI 9) in the medial aspect of the lower leg. Then it goes upward to the abdomen along the medial aspect of the lower limbs, meeting the Spleen Channel of Foot-Taiyin there. Then it runs to the costal region and meets the Liver Channel of Foot-Jueyin. From there, it goes upward further, reaching the throat and meets with the Ren Channel at Tiantu (RN 22) and Lianquan (RN 23) in the neck.

(8) The Yangwei Channel: This channel comes out from Jinmen (GB 63) of the Bladder Channel of Foot-Taiyang Below the external malleolus. Then it goes upward along the lateral aspect of the lower limbs together with the Gallbladder Channel of Foot-Shaoyang. Passing through the lateroposterior region of the trunk, it goes upward along the posterior end of the axillary fossa to the shoulder, where it continues to go upward to the neck and the retroauricular region. Then it goes anteriorly to the forehead and then to the nape, meeting with the Du Channel at Fengfu (DU 16) and Yamen (DU 15).

3. The branches of the twelve regular channels

The branches of the twelve regular channels are the portions of the twelve regular channels which travel to the depth of the body cavities.

Most of the branches of the twelve regular channels come out from their related channels above the knees or elbows, then they enter the thoracic and abdominal cavities. The branches of the Yang channels communicate with the Zang-Fu organs that their corresponding channels pertain to or connect with, and emerge in the nape or head. The branches of the Yang channels enter their corresponding channels and those of the Yin channels enter the Yang channels interior-exteriorly related with their corresponding channels. The branches of the Bladder Channel of Foot-Taiyang and the Kidney Channel of Foot-Shaoyin separate from their corresponding channels in the popliteal fossa, enter the body cavity to connect with the Kidney and the Bladder, emerge in the nape and enter their related Yang channel. The branches of the Gallbladder Channel of Foot-Shaoyang and the Liver Channel of Foot-Jueyin come out from their corresponding channels in the lower limbs, go upward to the public hairy region. enter the body cavity to connect with the Gallbladder and the Liver and then go upward to the eye system where they enter the Gallbladder Channel of Foot-Shaoyang. The branches of the Stomach Channel of Foot-Yangming and the Splenn Channel of Foot-Taiyin separate from their corresponding channels in the hip, then enter the body cavity to connect with the Spleen and the Stomach , and goes upward to the ala nasi to enter the Stomach Channel of Foot-Yangming. The branches of the Small Intestine Channel of Hand-Taiyang and the Heart Channel of Hand-Shaoyin come out from their corresponding channels in the axillary fossa, then enter the body cavity to connect with the Heart and the Small Intestine, and after that they go up to the inner canthus to enter the Small Intestine Channel of Hand-Taiyang. The branches of the Triple-Jiao Channel of Hand-Shaoyang and the Pericardium Channel of Hand-Jueyin enter the thoracic cavity to connect with the triple-Jiao and the Pericardium after separating from their corresponding channels, then they go upward to the retroauricular region to enter the Triple-Jiao Channel of Hand-Shaoyang. The branches of the Large Intestine Channel of Hand-Yangming and the Lung Channel of Hand-Taiyin connect with the Lung and the Large Intestine in the body cavity after separating from their corresponding regular channels, then they go upward to the supraclavicular fossa to enter the Large Intestine Channel of Hand-Yangming.

The branches of the twelve regular channels have the function of strengthening the connections among Zang-Fu organs and the connections among channels and other parts of the body, and extending the treatment areas of the acupints.

4. The fifteen major collaterals

The fifteen major collaterals refer to the major collaterals of the twelve regualr channels, the Ren and Du Channels and the splenic major collateral. They are named after the names of the acupoints where they originate.

Originating from the points of their original channels, the major collaterals of the twelve regular channels go to the channels interior-exteriorly related to the original channels, so they can extend the channels' distribution. The major collateral of the Du Channel starts from Changqiang (DU 1) and is distributed over the head, then it branches off into two parts and enter the Bladder Channel of Foot-Taiyin on the bilateral side of the head. The major collateral of the Ren Channel, after separating from Jiuwei (RN 15), is distributed over the abdomen. The splenic major collateral separates from Dabao (SP 21) and is distributed over the costal region. Of the collaterals of the whole body, the major collaterals are the large ones, while the superficial collaterals and the minute collaterals are the fine ones.

The major collaterals of the twelve regular channels have the function of strengthening the connection of the interior-exteriorly related channels. The major collateral of the Ren Channel communicates with Qi of channels in the abdomen, that of the Du Channel comminucates with Qi of channels in the back, and the splenic major collateral communicates with Qi of channels in the costal region. The minute collaterals are extremely fine and are distributed all over the body, with sending Qi and Blood to support the tissues of whole body as their main functions.

5. The twelve muscular regions

The twelve muscular regions are the systems of the meridians in the tendons, muscles and joints where the Qi of the twelve regular channel accumulates. They serve as the peripheral parts affiliated to the twelve regular channels.

The distribution of the twelve muscular regions are about the same as that of the twelve regular channel in the superficials. But they all go from the extremeties of the four limbs to the head and trunk, are distributed over the superficials rather than going deeply

31

into the body cavity and tend to accumulate in the joints and skelte-
tion of the body cavity and accumulate in the joints and skeletion.
The muscular regions of the three Yang channels of foot originate
from the toes, go upward along the lateral aspect of the thigh and
accumulate in the zygomatic region; while those of the three Yin
channels of foot originate from the toes and go upward along the medial aspect of the thigh to accumulate in the external genitalia. The
muscular regions of the three Yang channels of hand originate from
the fingers and go upward to accumulate in the corner of forehead a-
long the lateral aspect of the upper arm; while those of the three
Yin channels of the hand originate from the fingers and go upward
to accumulate in the diaphragm along the medial aspect of the upper
arm.

The main functions of the muscular regions are to control the
bones and benefit the movements of joints to ensure the normal
movements of human body.

6. The twelve cutaneous regions

The twelve cutaneous regions are the skin areas classified in accordance with the distribution of twelve regular channels and their
collaterals in the superficies. They serve as both the areas reflecting
the functional activities of the twelve regular channels and the areas
where Qi of the collaterals are diffused. As they are located superficially, they function to defend the human body, and thus they may
be where the exogenous pathogens enter the human body and where
disease of the Zang-Fu organs and channels are reflected.

Distributing Laws of the Fourteen
Channels on the Superficial

The fourteen channels refer to the twelve regular channels and the
Du and Ren Channels. Their distribution on the superficials is: The
Yin channels of the six Zang organs (the Heart, the Liver, the

Spleen, the Lung, the Kidney and the Pericardium) are distributed in the medial aspect of the limbs or the chest and the abdomen, of which the three Yin channels of hand are distributed in the medial aspect of the arms, and that of the feet in the medial aspect of the legs. The Yang channels of the six Fu organs are disatributed over the lateral aspect of the limbs or the head, the face, the back and the lumbar region, of which the three Yang channels of hands are distributed over the lateral aspects of the hands, and those of the feet, in the lateral aspects of the feet. In the lateral aspects of limbs, the Yangming channels go in the anterior borders of the limbs, the Shaoyang channels in the middle line of the limbs, and the Taiyang channel in the posterior borders of the limbs; while in the medial aspect of the limbs, the Taiyin channels run in the anterior border, the Jueyin channels in the middle line and the Shaoyin channels in the posterior border (in the lower legs, the Jueyin channel goes in the anterior border and crosses with the Taiyin channel at a point 8 cun above the tip of the medial malleolus). The Ren Channel is distributed along the anterior midline, and the Du Channel along the posterior midline.

Physiological Functions of Meridians and Clinical Application of Meridian Theory

1. Physiological functions of the meridians

The meridians function to communicate and connect with the Zang-Fu organs and the limbs. The human body is composed of the Zang-Fu organs, the limbs, the bones, the sensory organs, the skin, the muscles and the tendons, as well as Qi, Blood and Body Fluid. They are closely related to each other in structures and coordinated with each other in functional activities through the communication and connection of the meridians.

The meridians also have the function of sending Qi and Blood to the whole body and fighting againgst invasion of exogenous pathogens. Qi and Blood, the material basis for life activities of human body, can be sent to nourish the Zang-Fu organs and tissues through the meridians to maintain the normal life activities. As meridians can both allow Qi and Blood to flow in them and help flow of the defensive Qi and the nutritive Qi, the defensive Qi, which flows outside the vessels, and the nutritive Qi, which flows within vessels, can be distributed to the whole body and play their effect of defending against invasion of pathogens. So the meridians also have the function of preventing invasion of exogenous pathogens and protecting the human body.

2. Clinical application of the meridian theory

(1) Illustrating pathological changes: The function of the meridian in preventing invasion of exogenous pathogens will be weakened when the Vital Qi is deficient and the pathogents are exuberant. In this case, if the superficies are attacked by a pathogen, the pathogen may enter from the exterior to the interior or from the shallow area to the deep area of human body through the meridians. Or the other way round, diseases of the Zang-Fu organs may be reflected on the superficial tissues or organs through the meridians. In addition, meridians also serve as the passageway for diseases tranmitting among the Zang-Fu organs, from the superficial tissues and organs to the internal organs or vice versa.

(2) Guiding diagnosis in the clinic: This is mainly manifested as the syndrome identification in accordance with the distribution of channels. Such methods of syndrome identification as syndrome identification in accordance with the meridians, that in accordance with the six "channels" and that in accordance with the Wei, Qi, Ying and Blood levels all take the meridian theory as their basis. Besides, the meridian theory may also be applied in observation of the colours, palpation of pulse and inquiring about patient's conditions. In recent years, some scholars made dianosis in accordance with ternderness, nodules and streak-likes substances emerging in the distributing route of channels or some points where Qi of meridian

accumulates, or in accordance with the changes of the skins in morphological feature, temperature and electric resistance.

(3) Guiding treatment with acupuncture-moxibustion: The acupuncture-moxibustion treatment is carried out by needling or moxibusting the acupoints to promote flow of Qi in the channels, restore and regulate the functional activities of the Zang-Fu organs and Qi and Blood. Clinically, points are usually selected on the basis of the syndrome identification in accordance with the distribution of channels, apart from the points selected adjacent to the diseased area. The so-called selection of points along the distribution of channels means to select the points of the diseased channel or the diseased organ that the channel pertains to or the related channels, which are usually located far away from the diseased area. In addition, padding with cutaneous needles on the skin or embedding of the endocutaneous needles in the skin are often adopted to treat diseases of the Zang-Fu organs and channels. because the cutaneous regions have a close relationship with the channels and Zang-Fu organs. Diseases of the muscular regions are mostly treated by using the local points, which is known as painful points as the selected points.

(4) Guiding drugs tropism: Drugs tropism means a drug can be adopted to treat diseases of a special channel, which is based on classifications of drugs in accordance with the meridian theory. In almost each department of traditional Chinese medicine, formulas composed by drugs are the main method to treat diseases. it is an important method to enhance the therapeutic effect by using the drugs petaining to the diseased channels in accordance with their channel tropism when the disease location is identified. The formation, development and maturity of the drugs tropism result from the application of the meridian theory in the treatment of diseases with drugs.

In brief, the meridian theory penetrates through the whole course of diagnosis and treatment of diseases in various departments of traditional Chinese medicine.

Acupointology

*T*he acupointology is a subject dealing with formation of the acupoint theory, location and action of the acupoints, relations of the acupoints with Zang-Fu organs and tissues and application of the acupoints in prevention and treatment of disease. It is an important part of the science of acupuncture-moxibustion. Generally speaking, it involves classification, names, meanings of the names, locations, locating methods, local anatomy, actions, indications, needling methods and contraindications of the acupoints.

Acupoint is where Qi of the Zang-Fu organs and meridians is transmitted to the exterior of the human body.

A General Introduction of Acupoints

1. Classification and nomenclature of the acupoints

The acupoints are usually classified as three groups: The acupoints of the channels, the extra acupoints and the Ah Shi points.

The acupoints of channels, also known as the acupoints of the fourteen channels, refer to the acupoints pertaining to the twelve regular channels and the Ren and Du Channels. They have definite locations, names and pertaining channels. Functionally, they are used to treat diseases concerning the channels, and are regarded as one of the places where disease of the fourteen channels and the Zang-Fu organs are reflected. So they serve as the main part of the acupoints. There are 361 identified acupoints of channels in number by now.

The extra acupoints are the acupoints having definite names and locations but having hot been attributed to the fourteen channels. They usually have some special therapeutic effects on diseases.

The Ah Shi Points indicate the points with ternderness on palpation. They have not definite names and definite locations, and are mostly found in a localized area of the diseased part. Clinically, such points often produce ternderness and a feeling of comfort, hotness or aching. Be sure not to confuse the acupoints of channels or the extra acupoints selected based on their ternder response in treatment of disease with the Ah Shi points.

Names of the acupoints are an important component part of the terminology of the science of acupuncture-moxibustion. They are cosley related to the theory of TCM, the ancient Chinese philosophy, the ancient astronomy, the ancient geography, the traditional music instrument, the architecture as well as features of natural things. This is an evidence that the science of acupuncture-moxibustion has been constantly absorbing and applying the scientific achievements at different times in its historical development. As each acupoint has its special background, knowing the concrete meanings of the names of an acupoint can help to summarize the precious heritage of acupuncture-moxibustion and promote the development of the science of acupuncture-moxibustion. With the popularization of acupuncture-moxibustion, academic exchange is becoming more and more frequent. In December, 1982, the World Health Organization Regional Office for the Western Pacific organized a meeting in Manila and discussed the scheme for standard acupoint nomenclature, according to which the nomenclature of an acupoint should include three parts: the alphabetic code, Chinese pinyin and the Chinese characters of the acupoint. This has actually promoted the popularizaion and development of acupuncture-moxibustion in different countries of the world.

2. Therapeutic effects of the acupoints

This is mainly manifested as the following three aspects.

(1)Treating the disease around the acupoints: This is a common point of the therapeutic effects of all the acupoints. All the acupoints can be used to treat dieases in the area where the acupoints are situated or the diseases of the adjacent tissues and organs of the acupoints. For example, Jingming (BL 1), situated in the eye region, can be adopted to treat diseases of the eyes.

(2) Treating the diseases far away from the acupoints: This is a basic law of the therapeutic effects of the acupoints of channels. The acupoints of the fourteen channels, especially those of the twelve regular channels located below the knees and elbows, can be used not only to treat diseases of the areas where the points are located, but also to treat diseases of the Zang-Fu organs and tissues which are far away from the areas where the acupoints are located, since the pertaining channels of the acupoints pass through them. Some acupoints may even be employed to treat diseases of the whole body. For example, Hegu (LI 4) has a therapeutic effect on diseases of the hand or wrist where the point is located, diseases of the head and face which are distal to the hand, and such diseases involving the whole body such as fever caused by exogenous pathogens.

(3) Special therapeutic effects: Clinical practice has proved that a favorable double-way regulatory effect can be obtained by needling some acupoints in accordance with the different states of the human body. For example, needling Tianshu (ST 25) may prevent feces from discharging too frequently in the case of diarrhea and prevent feces from discharging rarely in the case of constipation. Besides, the therapeutic effect of the acupoints may be specific to some diseases. For example, Dazhui (DU 14) has a specific effect of reducing fever; Zhiyin (BL 67) has a specific effect of correcting the fetal position, etc.

To summarize, the therapeutic effects of the acupoints of the fourteen channels can be generalized as that an acupoint can treat diseases of the channel it pertains to, the acupoints of the interior-exteriorly related channels can be used exchangeably to treat diseases of these channels, and the acupoints adjacent to each other can be used jointly to treat diseases of the area where these acupoints are located.

3. Method to locate the acupoints

Clinically, the therapeutic effect is closely related to whether the acupoints are correctly located or not. So, it is very important to master the method to locate the acupoints in order to locate the acupoints correctly.

(1) Bone-length measurement: This is a method to measure the length and width of the different parts of the human body with the length of a bone as the proportional unit of the body in order to locate acupoints. It is a fundamental method to locate the acupoints. The follows are an introduction to the length of the different parts of the human body measured with this method.

① Head and face: The line connecting the midpoint of the anterior hairline and the midpoint of the posterior hairline is 12 cun, used to determine the longitude distance of the acupoints on the head; and the line connecting the left and the right corners of the hairline is 9 cun, used to measure the horizontal distance of the acupoints of the anterior part of the head; the line connecting the bilateral mastoid processes is 9 cun, used to determine the horizontal distance of the acupoints on the pasterior part of the head.

② The trunk: The line connecting the midpoint of the junction of the sternum and the xiphoid and the unmbilicus is 8 cun, used to determine the longitude distance of the acupoints in the upper abdomen; the line connecting the umbilicus and the upper border of the pubic syphysis is 5 cun, used to determine the longitude distance of the acupoints in the lower abdomen; the line connecting the bilateral nipples is 8 cun, used to determine the horizontal distance of the acupoints in the chest and abdomen; the line connecting the upper end of the axillary fossa and the free end of the 11th rib is 12 cun, used to determine the longitude distance of the acupoints in the costal region; the line connecting the medial border of the scapula and the posterior midline is 3 cun, used to determine the horizontal distance of the acupoints on the back and the lumbar region.

③ The upper limbs: The line connecting the anterior end of the axillary crease and the transverse crease of the elbow is 9 cun, used to determine the longitude distance of the acupoints in the upper arms; the line connecting the transverse crease of the elbow and the transverse crease of the wrist is 12 cun, used to determine the longitude distance of the acupoints in the forearms.

④ The lower limbs: The line connecting the upper border of the pubic syphysis and the upper border of the internal epicondyle of the femur is 18 cun, used to determine the longitude distance of the acupoints in the medial aspect of the thigh; the line connecting the internal epicondyle of the tibia and the tip of the medial malleolus is 13 cun, used to determine the longitude distance of the acupoints in the medial aspect of the lower leg; the line connecting the great trochanter of the femur and the transverse crease of the popliteal fossa is 19, used to determine the longitude distance of the acupoints in the postero-lateral aspect of the thigh; the line connecting the transverse crease of the popliteal fossa with the tip of the external malleolus is 16 cun, used to determine the longitude distance of the acupoints in the lateroposterior aspect of the lower leg.

(2) The superficial anatomic marks: This is a method to locate acupoints by means of the anatomical marks on the surface of the human body. The superficial anatomical marks can be classified as two types: The fixed marks which are not influenced by the human activities, such as the umbilicus; and the mobile marks, which indicate the foramen, depression or crease that appears when the joints, muslces and skin do voluntary movements. For example, Houxi (SI 3) can be located at the posterior end of the metacarpal crease when a fist is made.

(3) Simple method: This is a simple and convenient method to locate acupoints. For example, Lieque (LU 7) can be localized at where the tip of the index finger touches when the parts between the thumb and the index finger of both hand cross each other with the index fingers extending naturally.

(4) Finger proportional unit: This is a method to locate the acu-

points with the length of finger as a measuring unit, which is applicable to locating the points on the four limbs and the back. The commonly used finger proportional units are three kinds: The proportional unit with the middle finger as a standard, which means the distance between the two radial ends of the crease of the middle bone of the middle finger is taken as one cun; the proportional unit with the breadth of the closed four fingers as a standard, which means that the width passing through the crease of the middle metacarpal joint of the index finger when the four fingers are drawn close is taken as one cun; and the proportional unit with the thumb as a standard, which means the length of the interphalangeal joint of the thumb is taken as one cun.

4. Specific acupoints

Specific acupoints refer to a number of acupoints with specific therapeutic effects and names.

(1) The Five Shu-points: This is a collective term for the Jing-Well points, the Ying-Spring point, the Shu-Stream point, the Jing-River points and the He-Sea points of the twelve regular channels located below the knees and elbows. They are located from the extremities to the elbow or the knee in order. These points are so named because the flow of Qi in the channels resembles water flow in nature. Clinically, the Jing-Well point is usually used to treat mental diseases; the Ying-Spring point is used to treat febrile diseases; the Shu-Stream point is used to treat heavy sensation of the body and arthralgia; the Jing-River point is used to treat cough, asthma and disorders of the throat; and the He-Sea point is used to treat diseases of the six Fu organ, especially those of the gastrointestinal tract.

(2) The Yuan-Primary points: These points are where the primorial Qi passes and stagnates. Each of the twelve regular channels has a Yuan-Primary point on the limbs. The Yuan-Primary points have the function of correcting the Excess or Deficiency of the diseases of their pertaining channel, so they are very important in diagnosis and treatment of diseases of the Zang-Fu organs and channels.

(3) The Luo-Connecting points: Each collateral has a point in

which it separates from the channel. This point is known as the Luo-Connecting point. The Luo-Connecting points of the twelve regular channels are all located below the knees and elbows. Jiuwei (RN 15), the Luo-Connecting point of the Ren Channel, is situated in the abdomen; Changqiang (DU 1), the Luo-Connecting point of the Du Channel, is located in the sacral region; and Dabao (SP 21), the Luo-Connecting point of the splenic major collateral; is located in the costal region. So, there are 15 Luo-Connecting points in number. The Luo-Connecting points have the function of linking up the two channels interior-exteriorly related. Therefore, they can be adopted to treat disease of its pertaining collateral, as well as diseases of the interior-exteriorly related channels concerning the acupoints.

(4) The Xi-Cleft points: These refer to the places where the Qi of each meridian accumulates in the depth, most of which are located below the knees and elbows of the limbs. Each of the twelve regular channel, the Yinqiao Channel, the Yangqiao Channel, the Yinwei Channel and the Yangqiao Channel, has a Xi-Cleft point, and clinically, the Xi-Cleft point is mainly adopted to treat the acute diseases of the areas that the channel that the acupoint pertains to passes by and the acute diseases of the related Zang-Fu organs. The Xi-Cleft points of the Yin channels are mostly used to treat disorders of the Blood. For example, Kongzui (LU 6) can treat coughing blood. The Xi-Cleft points of the Yang channels can treat acute pains. For example, Waiqiu (GB 36) can be adopted to treat pain in the neck and nape.

(5) The Back-Shu points: These are the acupoints where the Qi of Zang-Fu organs is diffused on the back or lumbar region. They are located from the upper to the lower corresponding to the different locations of the different Zang-Fu organs in the first line distal to the anterior midline of the Bladder Channel of Foot-Taiyang, and are named after their corresponding Zang-Fu organs. They can be adopted to treat the diseases of both their corresponding Zang-Fu organs and the five sensory organs, the nine orifices, the skin, the muscle, the tendon and the bones related to the Zang-Fu organs.

For example, Ganshu (UB 18) can be used to treat Liver disease, eye disease and convulsion of the tendons. Compared with the Front-Mu points, the Back-Shu points are more frequently adopted to treat diseases of a Yin nature.

(6) The Front-Mu points: These are the acupoints where Qi of Zang-Fu organs accumulates in the chest and abdomen, which pertain to the six Zang organs and the six Fu organs respectively, so there are 12 Front-Mu points in all. The Front-Mu points may be located in their pertaining channels or in other channels, and they are often employed to treat diseases of their related organs. Compared with the Back-Shu points, the Front-Mu points are mostly chosen to treat diseases of a Yang nature.

(7) The eight confluential points: The eight confluential points are the acupoints where the essence Qi of Zang organs, the Fu organs, the Qi, the Blood, the tendon, the vessel, the bone and the marrow converge. Physiologically, they are closely related to the above mentioned Zang-Fu organs and tissues. Clinically, the eight confluential points are mainly used to treat diseases of the Zang organs, diseases of the Fu organs, disorder of Qi, disorder of Blood, diseases of the tendons, diseases of the vessels, diseases of the bones and diseases of the marrow respectively. For example, Juegu (GB 39), the confluential point of marrow, can be used to treat diseases of the bone marrow and the brain.

(8) The eight crossing points: The eight points connecting the eight extraordinary channels and the twelve regular channels are known as the eight crossing points, which are all located below the knees or the elbows. As Qi of the eight extraordinary channels and that of the twelve regular channel communicates with each other through the eight crossing points, the eight crossing points can be used to treat both the disease of the extraordinary channels and the regular channels they connect with. For example, Gongsun (SP 4), which communicates with the Chong Channel, can be adopted to treat diseases of the Spleen Channel of Foot-Taiyin and diseases of the Chong Channel, etc.

(9) The lower confluent points: These refer to the six points

where Qi of the three Yang channels of both hands and feet and that of the six Fu organs communicates with that of the three Yang channels of feet, which are mainly distributed around the knees. They serve as the main points to treat diseases of the six Fu organs. For example, Zusanli (ST 36) can be used to treat stomachache, and Shangjuxu (ST 37) can be used to treat dysentery, etc.

(10) The crossing points: These refer to the points by which two or more channels cross or converge, which are mainly located in the head and trunk. They can treat both the diseases of their pertaining channels and the diseases of the channels they cross. For example, Dazhui (DU 14), an acupoint of the Du Channel, is where the three Yang channels of both hands and feet meet, so it can be adopted to treat diseases of the Du Channel as well as diseases of all the Yang channels, or even diseases of the whole body.

Commonly Used Acupoints of the Fourteen Channels

1. The acupoints on the head and neck

(1) Shenting (DU 24):

Location: On the head, 0.5 cun directly above the midpoint of the anterior hairline.

Actions and indications: To fresh the mind, restore consciousness, and calm the mind; indicated for neurosis, schizophrenia, epilepsy, cerebrovascular diseases, common cold, rhinitis, conjunctivitits, etc.

Manipuation: Puncture 0.5-1 cun, or pricking to cause bleeding. Moxibustion is applicabble.

(2) Shangxing (DU 23):

Location: On the head, 1 cun directly above the midpoint of the naterior hairline.

Actions and indications: To dispel Wind and clear awar Heat, rest the Heart and remove onstruction from orifices; indicated for headache, dizziness, rhinitis, epistaxis, conjunctivititis, etc.

Manipulations: Puncture 0. 5-1 cun. Moxibustion is applicable.

(3) Baihui (DU 20):

Location: On the head, 5 cun above the midpoint of the anterior hairline, or at the midpoint of the line connecting the bilateral ear apex.

Actions and indications: To lift Yang, treat prostration, remove obstruction from the orifice and rest the mind; indicated for headache, dizziness, prolapse of retum, prolapse of uterus, schizophrenia, epilepsy and cerebrovascular diseases.

Manipulations: Puncture 0. 5-1 cun. Moxibustion is applicable.

Notes: This is the crossing point of the Du Channel and the Bladder Channel of Foot-Taiyang.

(4) Fengfu (DU 16):

Location: On the nape, 1 cun directly above the midpoint of the posterior hairline, directly below the external occipital protuberance, in the depression between the bilateral trapezius muscles.

Actions and indications: To dispel Wind and clear away Heat, restore consciousness and remove obstruction from the orifice; indicated for pharynitis, acute or chronic bronchitis, bronchial asthma, cerebrovascular diseases and hiccup.

Manipulations: Puncture vertically 0. 5-1 cun. Moxibustion is applicable.

Notes: Needle should be inserted slowly, and strong rotating, twisting, lifting and inserting manipulations must be avoided.

(5) Yamen (DU 15):

Location: On the nape, 0. 5 cun directly above the midpoint of the posterior hairline, below the 1st cervical vertebra.

Actions and indications: To treat dumb, remove obstruction from the orifice, clear away Heat from the Heart and calm the mind; used to treat cerebrovascular diseases, hysteria, epilepsy, schizophrenia, cerebral agenesis, deafness, dumb, neurologic headache, hoarseness, aphasia, epistaxis, injury of the soft tissues of the neck, cer-

45

vical spondylopathy.

Manipulation: Puncture 0. 5-1 cun slowly toward the mandible. Moxibustion with moxa cone is forbidden.

Notes: The needle must be inserted slowly and be sure not to puncture toward the tip of the nose. The depth of puncture should be less than 1. 5 cun, and once patient has a feeling of electric shock, the needle should be withdrawn at once.

(6) Tongtian (BL 7):

Location: On the head, 4 cun directly above the midpoint of the anterior hairline and 1. 5 cun lateral to the midline.

Actions and indications: To clear away Heat, dispel Wind and remove obstruction from collaterals and orifices, used to treat cerebrovascular diseases, trigeminal neuralgia, spasm of the facial muslces, facial paralysis, rhinitis, dysosmia, nasal sinusitis, bronchitis and bronchial asthma.

Manipulation: Puncture subcutaneously 0. 3-0. 5 cun. Moxibustion is applicable.

(7) Toulinqi (GB 15):

Location: On the head, 0. 5 cun within the hairs directly above the pupil, at the midpoint of the line connecting Shenting (DU 24)) and Touwei (ST 8).

Actions and indications: To clear away Heat from the head, improve eyesights, tranquilize and sedate the mind; used to treat headache, ametropia, cerebrovascular diseases and infantile convulsion.

Manipulation: Puncture subcutaneously 0. 5-1 cun. Moxibustion is applicable.

(8) Jiaosun (SJ 20):

Location: On the head, above the ear apex within the hairline.

Actions and indications: To clear away Heat, dispel Wind, subdue swelling and relieve pain; indicative for mumps, toothache, keratitis, retinal hemorrhage, optic neuritis, otitis media, tinnitus and deafness.

Manipulation: Puncture 0. 3-0. 5 cun subcutaneously. Moxibustion is applicable.

(9) Yifeng (SJ 17):

Location: Posterior to the lobule of the ear, in the depression between the mostoid process and the mandible.

Actions and indications: To remove obstructions from orifice, improve hearing, dispel Wind and purge Heat; indicated for headache, deafness, tinnitus, otitis media, toothache, facial paralysis, inflammation of the mandibular articulation, mumps, tuberculosis of the cervical lymph nodes, hiccup, etc.

Manipulation: Puncture perpendicularly 0. 5-1. 5 cun. Moxibustion is applicable.

Notes: This point is the crossing point of the Triple-Jiao Channel of Hand-Shaoyang and the Gallbladder Channel of Foot-Shaoyang.

(10) Fengchi (GB 20):

Location: On the nape, below the occipital bone, at the level of Fengfu (DU 16), in the depression between the upper end of the sternocleidomastoid and the trapezius muscles.

Actions and indications: To expel Wind, reduce fever, improve eyesights and remove obstructions from orifices; indicated for hypertension, cerebrovascular diseases, neurosis, Meniere's syndrome, common cold, tinnitus, deafness, stiff neck and pain in the heel.

Manipulation: Puncture 0. 8-1. 2 cun obliquely toward the tip of nose, or puncture through the point to Fengfu (DU 16) subcutaneously. Moxibustion is applicable.

Notes: This is the crossing point of the Gallbladder Channel of Foot-Shaoyang and the Yangwei Channel.

(11) Jingming (BL 1):

Location: On the face, in the depression slightly above the corner of the inner canthus.

Actions and indications: To dispel Wind, clear away Heat, nourish the Kidney and improve the eyesights; indicated for myopia, optic neuritis, atrophy of the optic nerve, glaucoma, pigmentary degeneration of the retina, conjunctivitis, keratis, hiccup, enuresis, diabetes insipidus, sciatica, and acute lumbar sprain.

Manipulation: Ask patient to shut his eyes. With the left hand mildly pushing the patient's eyeball laterally to fix it, the doctor punctures 0. 1-1 cun perpendicularly and slowly. No rotating, twisting, lifting and inserting manipulations are suggested. When the needle is withdrawn, press the hole for 1-2 minutes to avoid bleeding.

Notes: This is the crossing point of the Small Intestine Channel of Hand-Taiyang, the Bladder Channel of Foot-Taiyang, the Stomach Channel of Foot-Yangming, the Yinqiao Channel and the Yangqiao Channel.

(12) Sibai (ST 2):

Location: On the face, directly below the pupil, in the depression of the infraorbital foroman.

Actions and indications: To dispel Wind, improve eyesights, clear away Heat and activate Blood flow in the collaterals; indicated for trigeminal neuralgia, spasm of the facial muscles, facial paralysis, nasal sinusitis, myopia, conjunctivitis, keratitis, biliary ascariasis.

Manipulation: Puncture 0. 3-0. 5 cun perpendicularly or downward obsliquely.

(13) Yingxiang (LI 20):

Location: In the nasalabial groove, beside the midpoint of the lateral border of the nasal ala.

Actions and indications: To remove obstruction from the nose and dispel Wind; indicated for acute or chronic rhinitis, nasal sinusitis, epistaxis, facial paralysis, biliary ascariasis and constipation.

Manipulation: Puncture 0. 3-0. 5 cun obliquely or subcutaneously. Moxibustion with scar formation should be avoided.

Notes: This is the crossing point of the Large Intestine Channel of Hand-Yangming and the Stomach Channel of Foot-Yangming.

(14) Shuigou (DU 26):

Location: On the face, at the junction of the upper third and the middle third of the philtrum.

Actions and indications: To dispel Wind, restore consciousness, promote Blood flow in the channels and remove Blood Stasis from the collaterals; indicated for shock, coma, heat-stroke, epilepsy, hysteria, car-sick, boat-sick and acute lumbar sprain.

Manipulation: Puncture upward obliquely 0.3-0.5 cun. Moxibustion is applicable.

Notes: This is the crossing point of the Du Channel, the Large Intestine Channel of Hand-Yangming and the Stomach Channel of Foot-Yangming.

(15) Dicang (ST 4):

Location: On the face, beside the mouth angle, directly below the pupil.

Actions and indications: To expel Wind, support vital Qi, promote Blood flow in the channels and remove obstructiuons from the collaterals; indicated for facial paralysis, spasm of the facial muscles and trigeminal neuralgia.

Manipulation: Puncture toward Jiache (ST 6) subcutaneously 1-2 cun. Moxibustion is applicable.

(16) Jiache (ST 6):

Location: On the cheek, one finger breadth (middle finger) anterior and superior to the mandibular angle, in the depression where the masseter muscle is prominent when chewing.

Actions and indications: To calm Wind, clear away Heat, help open mouth and remove Blood Stasis from collaterals; indicated for facial paralysis, spasm of the facial muscles, trigeminal neuralgia, pulpitis and pericoronitis.

Manipulation: Puncture perpendicularly 0.3-0.5 cun or subcutaneously 0.5-1 cun. Moxibustion is applicable.

(17) Xiaguan (ST 7):

Location: On the face, anterior to the ear, in the depression of the zygomatic arc and the mandibular notch.

Actions and indications: To remove obstruction from the ear, promote Blood flow in the collaterals, dispel Wind and regulate flow of Qi; indicated for dysfunction of the tempo-mandibular joint, dislocation of the mandibular articulation, facial paralysis, trigeminal neuralgia, tinnitus, deafness, otitic dizziness and toothache.

Manipulation: Puncture perpendicularly 0.5-1 cun. Moxibustion is applicable.

(18) Tinggong (SI 19):

Location: On the face, anterior to the tragus and posterior to the mandibular condyloid process, in the depression found when the mouth is open.

Actions and indications: To disperse Qi in the ear, rest the Heart and tranquilize the mind; indicated for tinnitus, deafness, otitis externa and locked jaw.

Manipulation: Puncture perpendicularly 0.5-1 cun. Moxibustion is applicable.

Notes: This is the crossing point of the Triple-Jiao Channel of Hand-Shaoyang, the Gallbladder Channel of Foot-Shaoyang and the Small Intestine Channel of Hand-Taiyang.

(19) Chengjiang (RN 24):

Location: On the face, in the depression at the midpoint of the mentolabial sulcus.

Actions and indications: To relax tendons, dispel Wind, tranquilize the mind and promote production of Body Fluid; indicated for facial paralysis, bleeding and swollen gums, aphasia and diabetes.

Manipulation: Puncture subcutaneously 1-1.5 cun. Moxibustion is applicable.

Notes: This is the crossing point of the Ren Channel and the Stomach Channel of Foot-Yangming.

(20) Lianquan (RN 23):

Location: On the neck and the anterior midline, above the laryngeal protuberance, in the depression above the upper border of hyoid bone.

Actions and indications: To benefit the throat and tongue and regulate flow of Qi; indicated for sublingual swelling and pain, paralysis of the muscle of tongue, laryngnitis, tonsilitis, pharyngitis, lallation, dumb due to deafness, bronchitis and bronchial asthma.

Manipulation: Puncture 0.5-1 cun obliquely toward the root of the tongue. Moxibustion is applicable.

Notes: This is the crossing point of Yinwei Channel and the Ren Channel.

(21) Renying (ST 9):

Location: On the neck, beside the laryngeal protuberance, and on

50

the anterior border of sternocleidomastoid muscle where the pulsation of the common carotid artery is palpable.

Actions and indications: To promote Blood flow in the channels, regulate flow of Qi, dissipate nodules and relieve asthma; indicated for hypertension, hypotension, headache, trigeminal neuralgia, glaucoma, pharyngitis, tonsilitis, laryngitis, diseases of the vocal fold, goiter, hyperthroidism, bronchial asthma, Raynaud's disease, cardiac neurosis and cerebrovascular diseases.

Manipulation: Puncture 0. 3-0. 8 cun perpendicularly. Be sure to avoid puncturing the common carotid artery.

(22) Tianchuang (SI 16):

Location: On the lateral side of the neck, posterior to sternocleidomastoid muscle and Futu (LI 18), at the level of the pharyngeal protuberance.

Actions and indications: To soothe flow of the Lung Qi, relieve asthma, treat hoarseness and relieve cough; indicated for pharyngitis, laryngitis, tonsilitis, aphasia, acute or chronic bronchitis, bronchial asthma, bronchoectasis, pneumonia, goiter, esophagitis, gastritis, hepatitis and hiccup.

Manipulation: Puncture perpendicularly 0. 2 cun first, then puncture 0. 5-1 cun downward close to the posterior aspect of the sternum. Moxibustion is applicable.

Notes: The angle and depth of puncturing mentioned above must be strictly followed to avoid injury to the lung and the related arteries or veins. This point is the crossing point of the Yinwei Channel and the Ren Channel.

2. The acupoints on the trunk

(1) Shanzhong (RN 17):

Location: On the chest and the anterior midline, at the level of the 4th intercostal space and the midpoint of the line connecting the bilateral nipples.

Actions and indications: To soothe flow of Qi in the chest, relieve stagnation of Qi, relieve asthma and cough; indicated for bronchitis, bronchial asthma, pneumonia, angina pectoris, intercostal neuralgia, esophgitis, mastitis and hypogalactia.

Manipulation: Puncture subcutaneously 1-1. 5 cun. Moxibustion is applicable.

Notes: This is the Front-Mu point of the Pericardium as well as one of the eight confluential points where Qi converges.

(2) Jiuwei (RN 15):

Location: In the upper abdomen, on the anterior midline, 1 cun below the xiphosternal synchondrosis.

Actions and indications: To soothe flow of Qi in the chest, benefit the diaphragm, rest the Heart and tranquilize the mind; indicated for bronchial asthma, emphysema, intercostal neuralgia, angina pectoris, spasm of the diaphragm, gastritis, gastric ulcer, laryngitis, tonosilitis, pharyngitis, epilepsy, hysteria and schizophrenia.

Manipulation: Puncture 0. 5-1 cun subcutaneously. Moxibustion is applicable.

Notes: This is the Luo-Connecting point of the Ren Channel.

(3) Juque (RN 14):

Location: In the upper abdomen, on the anterior midline, 6 cun above the unbilicus.

Actions and indications: To soothe flow of Qi in the chest, remove retained food, clear away Heat from the Heart and calm the mind; indicated for bronchitis, bronchial asthma, pleuritis, angina pectoris, spasm of the diaphragm, hepatitis, gastritis, enteritis, epilepsy, schizophrenia, syncope and toxemia of pregnancy.

Manipulation: Puncture 1-1. 5 cun subcutaneously. Moxibustion is applicable.

Notes: This is the Front-Mu point of the Heart.

(4) Zhongwan (RN 12):

Location: In the upper abdomen, on the anterior midline, 4 cun above the centre of the umbilicus.

Actions and indications: To regulate the function of the Stomach, strengthen the Spleen, warm up Yang Qi in the Middle-Jiao and dissolve Dampness; indicated for gastritis, gastric ulcer, gastroptosis, gastrospasm, enteritis, dysentery, appendicitis, spasm of the diaphragm, cholecystitis, chronic hepatitis, constipation, bronchial asthma, cardiac diseases, sun-stroke, epilepsy and hysterica.

Manipulation: Puncture 0. 8-1. 5 cun perpendicularly. Moxibustion is applicable.

Notes: This is the Front-Mu point of the Stomach, one of the eight confluential points where Qi of the six Fu organs converges.

(5) Jianli (RN 11):

Location: In the upper abdomen, on the anterior midline, 3 cun above the umbilicus.

Actions and indications: To regulate the function of the Stomach, strengthen the Spleen, lower down upward adverse flow of Qi and induce diuresis; indicated for gastritis, neurogenic vomiting, indigestion, enteritis and nephritis.

Manipulation: Puncture 1-1. 5 cun perpendicularly. Moxibustion is applicable.

(6) Shenque (RN 8):

Location: In the middle abdomen or at the centre of the umbilicus.

Actions and indications: To warm up Yang, rescue patient from collapse, induce diuresis and relieve prostration; indicated for syncope, shock, acute cerebrovascular diseases, edema, enteritis, dysentery, constipation and inflammation of the urinary system.

Manipulation: Puncture is contraindicated. It is mostly treated with moxa cone with ginger and salt or with moxa stick.

(7) Qihai (RN 6):

Location: In the lower abdomen, on the anterior midline, 1. 5 cun below the umbilicus.

Actions and indications: To supplement the primordial Qi, warm up the Kidney and induce diuresis; indicated for collapse, angina pectoris, bronchial asthma, gastritis, constipation, frequent urination, enuresis, impotence, dysmenorrhea, irregular menstruation, amenorrhea, pelvic inflammation, dysfunctional uterine bleeding, lochiorrhea and general debility.

Manipulation: Puncture 0. 5-1 cun perpendicularly. Moxibustion is applicable.

Notes: This point has the effect of strengthening the body constitution, so it is considered to be an important point for health care.

(8) Guanyuan (RN 4):

Location: In the lower abdomen, on the anterior midline, 3 cun above the umbilicus.

Actions and indications: To strengthen the Kidney, consolidate the primordial Qi, warm up channel and dispel Cold; indicated for abdominal pain, diarrhea, enuresis, impotence, nephritis, urinary tract infection, irregular menstruation, dysmenorrhea, pelvic inflammation, dysfunctional uterine bleeding, sterility, lochiorrhea, cerebrovascular diseases and general weakness.

Manipulation: Puncture 0. 8-1. 2 cun perpendicularly. Moxibustion is applicable.

Notes: This point has an effect of strengthening the body constitution and is the Front-Mu point of the Small Intestine.

(9) Zhongji (RN 3):

Location: In the lower abdomen, on the anterior midline, 4 cun below the umbilicus.

Actions and indications: To tonify the Kidney, invigorate Yang Qi, regulate menstruation and stop leukorrhea; indicated for nephritis, urinary tract infection, irregular menstruation, pelvic inflammation, dysfunctional uterine bleeding, sterility, lochiorrhea, enuresis, nocturnal emission, impotence and premature ejaculation.

Manipulation: Puncture 0. 5-1 cun perpendicularly. Moxibustion is applicable.

Notes: This is the Front-Mu point of the Bladder, and the crossing point of the Ren Channel with the three Yin channels of feet.

(10) Tianshu (ST 25):

Location: In the middle abdomen, 2 cun lateral to the umbilicus.

Actions and indications: To regulate the function of the Stomach, regulate flow of Qi and strengthen the Spleen; indicated for acute gastroenteritis, dysentery, constipation, cholecystitis, hepatitis, nephritis, arthralgia, dysmenorrhea, uterine endometritis, dysfunctional uterine bleeding and infantile diarrhea.

Manipulation: Puncture 0. 5-1 cun perpendicularly. Moxibustion is applicable.

Notes: This is the Front-Mu point of the Large Intestine.

(11) Qimen (LR 14):

Location: In the chest, directly below the nipple, at the level of the 6th intercostal space, 4 cun lateral to the anterior midline.

Actions and indications: To relieve stagnation of the Liver Qi, strengthen the Spleen and clear away Heat; indicated for intercostal neuralgia, hepatitis, hepatauxe, cholecystitis, pleuritis, gastric neurosim, dysmenorrhea and mastitis.

Manipulation: Puncture 0. 5-1 cun subcutaneously. Moxibustion is applicable.

Notes: This is the Front-Mu point of the Liver.

(12) Riyue (GB 24):

Location: In the upper abdomen, directly below the nipple, at the level of the 7th intercostal space, 4 cun lateral to the anterior midline.

Actions and indications: To soothe flow of the Liver Qi, benefit the Gallbladder, resolve Dampness and regulate the function of the Middle-Jiao; indicated for gastritis, cholecystitis, hepatitis and intercostal neuralgia.

Manipulation: Puncture 0. 5-0. 8 cun obliquely or perpendicularly. Moxibustion is applicable.

Notes: This is the Front-Mu point of the Gallbladder.

(13) Tianzong (SI 11):

Location: In the scapular region, in the depression of the center of the subscapular fossa, and at the level of the 5th thoracic vertebra.

Actions and indications: To relax the tendons, promote Blood flow in the collaterals, purify and lower down the Lung Qi; indicated for periarthritis of the shoulder, injury of the soft tissues of shoulder and asthma.

(14) Tianzhu (BL 11):

Location: On the back, below the the spinous process of the 1st thoracic vertebra, 1. 5 cun lateral to the posterior midline.

Actions and indications: To clear away Heat, dispel Wind, strengthen the tendon and bones; indicated for common cold, laryngitis, bronchitis, bronchial asthma, hypertrophic spondylitis, rheumatic arthritis, stiff neck, cervical spondylopathy and stye.

Manipulation: Puncture 0. 5-0. 8 cun subcutaneously. Moxibustion is applicable.

Notes: One of the eight confluential points where bones converge. It is also the crossing point of the Small Intestine Channel of Hand-Taiyang and the Bladder Channel of Foot-Taiyang.

(15) Feishu (BL 13):

Location: On the back, below the spinous process of the 3rd thoracic vertebra, 1. 5 cun lateral to the posterior midline.

Actions and indications: To clear away Heat, relieve exterior syndrome, facilitate flow of the Lung Qi and regulate flow of Qi; indicated for common cold, bronchitis, bronchial asthma, pneumonia, emphysema, lung tuberculosis, lymphoid tuberculosis, pleuritis, nephritis, rheumatic arthritis and whooping cough.

Manipulation: Puncture 0. 5-1 cun perpendicularly. Moxibustion is applicable.

(16) Xinshu (BL 15):

Location: On the back, below the spinous process of the 5th cervical vertebra, 1. 5 cun lateral to the posterior midline.

Actions and indications: To activate Blood, regulate flow of Qi, clear away Heat from the Heart and tranquilize the mind; indicated for tachycardia, atrial fibrillation, angina pectoris, intercostal neuralgia, insomnia, forgetfulness, injury of the soft tissues of the back.

Manipulation: Puncture 0. 5-1 cun subcutaneously. Moxibustion is applicable.

(17) Ganshu (BL 18):

Location: On the back, below the spinous process of the 9th cervical vertebra, 1. 5 cun lateral to the posterior midline.

Actions and indications: To soothe flow of the Liver Qi, benefit the Gallbladder and relieve mental depression; indicated for ptosis of the eyelids, conjunctivitis, trachoma, glaucoma, night blindness, retinitis, lymphoid tuberculosis, intercostal neuralgia, hepatitis, cirrhosis of liver, cholelithiasis, cholecystitis, gastritis, dizziness, schizophrenia and hysterica.

56

Manipulation: Puncture 0.5-0.8 cun subcutaneously or obliquely. Moxibustion is applicable.

(18) Danshu (BL 19):

Location: On the back, below the spinous process of the 10th cervical vertebra, 1.5 cun lateral to the posterior midline.

Actions and indications: To benefit the Gallbladder, soothe the flow of the Liver Qi, regulate the function of the Stomach and lower down the upward adverse flow of Qi; indicated for cholecystitis, cholelithiasis, biliary ascariasis, hepatitis, cirrhosis of the liver, gastritis, peptic ulcer, insomnia and hysterica.

Manipulation: Puncture 0.5-0.8 cun obliquely. Moxibustion is applicable.

(19) Pishu (BL 20):

Location: On the back, below the spinous process of the 11th cervical vertebra, 1.5 cun lateral to the posterior midline.

Actions and indications: To strengthen the Spleen to control Blood, regulate the function of the Stomach and supplement Qi; indicated for gastritis, gastric ulcer, gastroptosis, indigestion, progressive muscular atrophy, anemia, enteritis, dysentery, hamefecia, irregular menstruation and dysfunctional uterine bleeding.

Manipulation: Puncture 0.5-0.8 cun obliquely. Moxibustion is applicable.

(20) Weishu (BL 21):

Location: On the back, below the spinous process of the 12th cervical vertebra, 1.5 cun lateral to the posterior midline.

Actions and indications: To regulate the function of the Stomach, strengthen the Spleen, aid digestion and remove Dampness; indicated for gastritis, gastric ulcer, indigestion, progressive muscular atrophy, enteritis, dysentery, hepatitis and diabetes.

Manipulation: Puncture 0.5-0.8 cun obliquely. Moxibustion is applicable.

(21) Sanjiaoshu (BL 22):

Location: In the lumbar region, below the spinous process of the 1st lumbar vertebra, 1.5 cun lateral to the posterior midline.

Actions and indications: To promote the function of the Triple-

Jiao, warm up Yang to dissolve Dampness; indicated for gastritis, enteritis, dysentery, constipation, nephritis, enuresis, nocturnal e-mission, edema, dizziness and insomnia.

Manipulation: Puncture 0. 5-1 cun perpendicularly. Moxibustion is applicable.

(22) Shenshu (BL 23):

Location: In the lumbar region, below the spinous process of the 2nd lumbar vertebra, 1. 5 cun lateral to the posterior midline.

Actions and indications: To nourish water, reduce the Fire and improve eyesight and the hearing; indicative for diseases of the urinary or the reproductive system, tinnitus, deafness, dizziness, insomnia, strain of the lumbar muscle and infantile diarrhea.

Manipulation: Puncture 0. 5-1 cun perpendicularly. Moxibustion is applicable.

(23) Dachangshu (BL 27):

Location: In the lumbar region, below the spinous process of the 4th lumbar vertebra, 1. 5 cun lateral to the posterior midline.

Actions and indications: To regulate the function of the gastrointestinal tract, promote flow of Qi and remove Dampness; indicated for indigestion, diarrhea, dysentery, intestinal obstruction, hemorrhoid, prolapse of rectum and lumbago.

Manipulation: Puncture 0. 8-1. 5 cun perpendicularly. Moxibustion is applicable.

(24) Xiaochangshu (BL 27):

Location: In the sacral region, at the level of the 1st posterior sacral foramen, 1. 5 cun lateral to the median sacral crest.

Actions and indications: To clear away Heat, remove Dampness, and regulate defecation and urination; indicated for enteritis, dysentery, diarrhea, pelvic inflammation and cytitis.

Manipulation: Puncture 0. 8-1. 2 cun perpendicularly. Moxibustion is applicable.

(25) Pangguangshu (BL 28):

Location: In the sacral region, at the level of the 2nd posterior sacral foramen, 1. 5 cun lateral to the median sacral crest.

Actions and indications: To clear away Heat, induce diuresis, and invigorate the Kidney Qi; indicated for diseases of the urinary or the reproductive system and neuralgia in the lumbar or the sacral region.

Manipulation: Puncture 0. 8-1. 2 cun perpendicularly. Moxibustion is applicable.

(26) Ciliao (BL 32):

Location: In the sacral region, medial and posterior to the posterosuperior illiac spine, just at the 2nd posterior sacral foramen.

Actions and indications: To tonify the Lower-Jiao, clear away Heat and remove Dampness; indicated for neuralgia in the sacral region and diseases of the urinary or the reproductive system.

Manipulation: Puncture 1-1. 5 cun perpendicularly. Moxibustion is applicable.

(27) Xialiao (BL 34):

Location: In the sacral region, medial and inferior to Zhongliao (BL 33), just at the 4th posterior sacral foramen.

Actions and indications: To tonify the Lower-Jiao, clear away Heat and remove Dampness; indicated for strain of the lumbar region, enteritis, dysentery, constipation, irregular menstruation, dysmenorrhea, leukorrhea, nocturnal emission, impotence, oliguria, enuresis and hernia.

Manipulation: Puncture 1-1. 5 cun perpendicularly. Moxibustion is applicable.

(28) Dazhui (DU 14):

Location: On the posterior midline, in the depression below the spinous process of the 7th cervical vertebra.

Actions and indications: To clear away Heat, supplement Qi, nourish Blood and tranquilize the mind; indicated for fever, sunstroke, malaria, schizophrenia, epilepsy, bronchitis, bronchial asthma, lung tuberculosis, emphysema, hepatitis, gematopathy, eczema and pain of the shoulder and the back.

Manipulation: Puncture 0. 5-1 cun obliquely downward. Moxibustion is applicable.

(29) Zhiyang (DU 19):

Location: On the back, on the posterior midline, in the depression below the spinous process of the 7th thoracic vertebra.

Actions and indications: To clear away Heat, remove Dampness, facilitate flow of the Lung Qi and relieve cough; indicated for bronchitis, bronchial asthma, intercostal neuralgia, hepatitis and cholecystitis.

Manipulation: Puncture 0. 5-1 cun upward obliquely. Moxibustion is applicable.

(30) Mingmen (DU 4):

Location: In the lumbar region, on the posterior midline, in the depression below the spinous process of the 2nd lumbar vertebra.

Actions and indications: To consolidate the essence, invigorate Yang, build up the primordial Qi and tonify the Kidney; indicated for lumbago, sprain of lumbar muscle, enuresis, nocturnal emission, impotence, irregular menstruation, leukorrhea, endometritis, pelvic inflammation, sciatica, sequele of poliomyelitis and nephritis.

Manipulation: Puncture 0. 5-1 cun perpendicularly. Moxibustion is applicable.

(31) Changqiang (DU 1):

Location: Below the tip of the coccyx, at the midpoint of the line connecting the anus and the tip of the coccyx.

Actions and indications: To nourish Yin, suppress Yang, supplement Qi and relieve prostration; indicated for hemorrhoids, prolapse of the rectum, eczema of the scrotum, diarrhea, schizophrenia and inducing abortion.

Manipulation: Puncture 1-1. 5 cun upward obliquely along the anterior aspect of the coccyx. Moxibustion is applicable.

Notes: This is the Luo-Connecting point of the Du Channel.

3. The acupoints of the upper limbs

(1) Shaoshang (LU 11):

Location: On the radial side of the distal segment of the thumb, 0. 1 cun from the corner of the nail.

Actions and indications: To clear away Heat, benefit throat, restore consciousness and remove obstructions from the orifice; indicated for laryngitis, tonsilitis, pharyngitis, bronchitits, bronchial asthma, pneumonia, mumps, epistaxis, aphasia, hiccup, coma and shock.

Manipulation: Puncture 0.1 cun perpendicularly or prick to let bleeding. Moxibustion is applicable.

Notes: This is the Jing-Well point of the Lung Channel of Hand-Taiyin.

(2) Taiyuan (LU 9):

Location: At the radial end of the transverse crease of the wrist where the pulsation of the radial artery is palpable.

Actions and indications: To supplement Qi, tranquilize the mind, relieve cough and asthma; indicated for tonsilitis, pneumonia, intercostal neuralgia, tachycardia, arthralgia around the wrist.

Manipulation: Puncture 0.3-0.5 cun perpendicularly. Avoid puncturing the radial artery, and moxibustion is applicable.

Notes: This is the Shu-Stream and Yuan-Source points of the Lung Channel of Hand-Taiyin. It is also one of the eight confluential points where the vessels converge.

(3) Lieque (LU 7):

Location: On the radial border of the forearm, proximal to the styloid process of radius, 1.5 cun above the crease of the wrist, between the brachioradial muscle and the tendon of the long abductor muscle of thumb.

Actions and indications: To expel Wind, dispel pathogen and regulate the function of the Ren Channel; indicated for diseases of the soft tissues of the wrist, deviation of the mouth and eyes, rigidity of the nape, epistaxis, laryngitis, bronchitis, enuresis and retetion of urine.

Manipulation: Puncture 0.5-0.8 cun upward obliquely. Moxibustion is applicable.

Notes: This is the Luo-Connecting point of the Lung Channel of Hand-Taiyin and one of the crossing point of the eight extraordinary channels, which communicates with the Ren Channel.

(4) Kongzui (LU 6):

Location: On the radial side of the palmar aspect of the forearm, on the line connecting Chize (LU 5) and Taiyuan (LU 9), 7 cun above the crease of the wrist.

Actions and indications: To clear away Heat and remove toxic substances, lower down the upward adverse flow of Qi and stop bleeding; indicated for headache due to common cold, laryngitis, bronchitis, lung tuberculosis, epistaxis, pain of the elbow and the forearm.

Manipulation: Puncture 0.8-1 cun perpendicularly. Moxibustion is applicable.

Notes: This is the Xi-Cleft point of the Lung Channel of Hand-Taiyin.

(5) Chize (LU 5):

Location: In the cubital crease, in the depression of the radial side of the tendon of biceps muscle of arm.

Actions and indications: To nourish Yin, moisten the Lung, stop cough and lower down upward adverse flow of Qi; indicated for common cold, laryngitis, pharyngitis, tonsilitis, bronchitis, acute gastroenteritis, mastitis, sprain of the lumbar muscle, sequele of cerebrovascular diseases, infantile convulsion and whooping cough.

Manipulation: Puncture 0.5-1 cun perpendicularly. Moxibustion is applicable.

Notes: This is the He-Sea point of the Lung Channel of Hand-Taiyin.

(6) Zhongchong (PC 9):

Location: At the centre of the tip of the middle finger.

Actions and indications: To restore Yang and rescue patient from collapse, relieve coma and promote Blood flow in the collaterals; indicated for angina pectoris, cerebral bleeding, shock, sun-stroke, collapse, hysteria, epilepsy, infantile convulsion, glossitis and infantile indigestion.

Manipulation: Puncture 0.1 cun superficially or prick to cause bleeding. Moxibustion is applicable.

Notes: This is the Jing-Well point of the Pericardium Channel of Hand-Jueyin.

(7) Laogong (PC 8):

Location: At the centre of the palm, between the 2nd and the 3rd metacarpal bones, but close to the latter, and in the part touching the tip of the middle-finger when a fist is made.

Actions and indications: To tranquilize the mind, lower down the upward adverse flow of Qi, clear away Heat from the Heart and relieve itching; indicated for coma in stroke, sun-stroke, angina pectoris, stomatitis, schizophrenia, hysteria, infantile convulsion, numbness of the fingers, hand sweating and tinea of the hand.

Manipulation: Puncture 0.5-0.8 cun. Moxibustion is applicable.

Notes: This is the Ying-Spring point of the Pericardium Channel of Hand-Jueyin.

(8) Daling (PC 7):

Location: At the midpoint of the crease of the wrist, between the tendons of long palmar muscle and radial flexor muscle of the wrist.

Actions and indications: To calm the mind, soothe flow of Qi in the chest and regulate the function of the Stomach; indicated for myocarditis, gastritis, tonsilitis, intercostal neuralgia, insomnia, epilepsy, schizophrenia, hysteria, disorders of the wrist and the soft tissues around it.

Manipulation: Puncture 0.5-0.8 cun perpendicularly. Moxibustion is applicable.

Notes: This is the Shu-Stream and the Yuan-Source point of the Pericardium Channel of Hand-Jueyin.

(9) Neiguan (PC 8):

Location: In the palmar side of the forearm, on the line connecting Quchi (LI 11) and Daling (PC 7), 2 cun above the crease of the wrist, between the tendons of long palmar muscle and the radial flexor muscle of the wrist.

Actions and indications: To soothe flow of Qi in the chest, regulate the function of the Stomach, tranquilize the mind and relieve palpiatation; indicated for angina pectoris, palpitation, chest pain, abdominal pain, stomachache, vomiting, spasm of diaphragm, epilepsy, insomnia, swelling and pain of throat and various kind of pains during operation.

Manipulation: Puncture 0.5-1 cun perpendicularly. Moxibustion is applicable.

Notes: This is the Luo-Connecting point of the Pericardium Channel of Hand-Jueyin, it is also one of the crossing points of the eight extraordinary channels which communicate with the Yinwei Channel.

(10) Quze (PC 3):

Location: In the cubital crease, at the ulnar border of the tendon of the biceps muscle of the arm.

Actions and indications: To regulate Qi and Blood, clear away Heat and relieve restlessness; indicated for angina pectoris, palpitation, common cold, vomiting due to gastritis, pain in the hand, elbow and forearm.

Manipulation: Puncture 1-1. 5 cun perpendicularly or prick to cause bleeding. Moxibustion is applicable.

Notes: This is the He-Sea point of the Pericardium Channel of Hand-Jueyin.

(11) Shaochong (HT 9):

Location: In the radial side of the distal segment of the little finger, 0. 1 cun from to the corner of nail.

Actions and indications: To calm the mind, fresh the brain, clear away Heat and tranquilize Wind; indicated for angina pectoris, palpitation, pleuritis, intercostal neuralgia, epilepsy and syncope.

Manipulation: Puncture 0. 1 cun superficially or prick to cause bleeding. Moxibustion is applicable.

Notes: This is the Jing-Well point of the Heart Channel of Hand-Shaoyin.

(12) Shenmen (HT 7):

Location: On the wrist, at the ulnar end of the crease of the wrist, in the depression of the radial side of the tendon of the ulnar flexor muscle of the wrist.

Actions and indications: To tranquilize the mind, support Vital Qi and eliminate pathogen; indicated for forgetfulness, insomnia, dream-disturbed sleep, palpitation, angina pectoris, hysteria, schizophrenia and epilepsy.

Manipulation: Puncture 0. 5-0. 8 cun perpendicularly. Moxibustion is applicable.

Notes: This is the Shu-Stream and Yuan-Source point of the

Heart Channel of Hand-Shaoyin.

(13) Yinxi (HT 6):

Location: In the palmar side of the forearm, in the radial border of the ulnar flexor muslce of the wrist, 0.5 cun above the crease of the wrist.

Actions and indications: To clear away Heat from the Heart, tranquilize the mind, consolidate the superficies and benefit the vocal fold; indicated for aphasia, epistaxis, hemetemesis, night sweating, angina, pectoris and epilepsy.

Manipulations: Puncture 0.5-0.8 cun. Moxibustion is applicable.

Notes: This is the Xi-Cleft point of the Heart Channel of Hand-Shaoyin.

(14) Tongli (HT 3):

Locations: When the elbow is flexed, this point is located at the midpoint of the line connecting the medial end of the cubital crease and the internal epicondyle of the femur.

Actions and indications: To open the orifices of the Heart, soothe flow of Qi in the chest and promote flow of Blood in the collaterals; indicated for lymphoid tuberculosis, headache, angina pectoris, pain in the hypochondriac region, shoulder pain, tremor of hands and paralysis of the lower limbs.

Manipulation: Puncture 0.5-1 cun perpendicularly. Moxibustion is applicable.

Notes: This is the He-Sea point of the Heart Channel of Hand-Shaoyin.

(15) Shaoze (SI 1):

Location: On the ulnar side of the distal segment of the little finger, 0.1 cun from the corner of the nail.

Actions and indications: To clear away Heat, promote discharge of milk, remove Blood Stasis and benefit orifices; indicated for headache, fever, syncope, laryngitis, hiccup, conjunctivitis, cataract, hypogalactia and mastitis.

Manipulation: Puncture 0.1 cun superficially or prick to cause to bleeding. Moxibustion is applicable.

Notes: This is the Jing-Well point of the Small Intestine Channel of Hand-Taiyang.

(16) Houxi (SI 3):

Location: At the junction of the white and red skin along the ulnar border of the hand, at the ulnar end of the distal palmar crease, proximal to the back of the metacarpophalangeal joint of the little finger when a hollow fist is made.

Actions and indications: To promote Blood flow in the collaterals, relieve mental depression, clear away Heat and treat malaria; indicated for headache, fever, stye, deafness, tinnitus, spasm of the facial muscle, stiff neck, hysteria, jaundice, malaria, night sweating, impetigo, urticaria, pain in the arm, leg or shoulder, and infantile convulsion.

Manipulation: Puncture 0. 5-2 cun perpendicularly. Moxibustion is applicable.

Notes: This is the Shu-Stream point of the Small Intestine Channel of Hand-Taiyang. It is also one of the eight crossing point of the eight exytraordinary channels which communicates with the Du Channel.

(17) Zhizheng (SI 7):

Location: On the ulnar side of the posterior surface of the forearm and on the line connecting Yanggu (SI 5) and Xiaohai (SI 8), 5 cun proximal to the dorsal crease of the wrist.

Actions and indications: To relieve exterior syndrome, clear away Heat, expel pathogen and relax muscles and tendons; indicated for common cold, headache, pain of tongue, diabetes and pain in the elbow and arm.

Manipulation: Puncture 0. 5-1 cun perpendicualrly. Moxibustion is applicable.

Notes: This is the Luo-Connecting point of the Small Intestine Channel of Hand-Taiyang.

(18) Guanchong (SJ 1):

Location: On the ulnar side of the distal segment of the ring finger, 0. 1 cun from the corner of the nail.

Actions and indications: To clear away Heat, relieve exterior syndrome and disperse flow of Qi in the Triple-Jiao; indicated for common cold, laryngitis, tonsilitis, conjunctivitis, optic neuritis, tinnitus,, deafness, periarthritis of the shoulder, cerebrovascular diseases and infantile convulsion.

Manipulation: Puncture 0. 1 cun obliquely to prick to cause bleeding. Moxibustion is applicable.

Notes: This is the Jing-Well point of the Triple-Jiao Channel of Hand-Shaoyang.

(19) Yemen (SJ 2):

Location: On the dorsum of the hand, between the 4th and the 5th fingers, at the junction of the white and red skin proximal to the margin of the web.

Actions and indications: To disperse Wind pathogen, regulate flow of Qi and improve hearing; indicated for headache, conjunctivitis, keratitis, tinnitus, deafness, toothache, mouth ulcer, tonsilitis, cervical spondylopathy, periarthritis of the shoulder, paralysis of the upper limb and malaria.

Manipulation: Puncture 0. 3-0. 5 cun obliquely. Moxibustion is applicable.

Notes: This is the Ying-Spring point of the Triple-Jiao Channel of Hand-Shaoyang.

(20) Zhongzhu (SJ 3):

Location: On the dorsum of the hand, proximal to the 4th metacapophalangeal joint, in the depresssion between the 4th and the 5th metacarpal bones.

Actions and indications: To clear away Heat, disperse pathogen, improve eyesights and benefit hearing; indicated for headache, conjunctivitis, optic neuritis, supraorbital neuralgia, tinnitus, deafness, Menere's syndrome, laryngitis, tonsilitis, spasm of the diaphragm, intercostal neuralgia, lumbago, periarthritis of the shoulder, paralysis of the upper limbs and inflammation of the phalangeal joint.

Manipulation: Puncture 0. 3-0. 5 cun perpendicularly. Moxibustion is applicable.

Notes: This is the Shu-Stream point of the Triple-Jiao Channel of Hand-Shaoyang.

(21) **Waiguan** (SJ 5):

Location: On the dorsal side of the forearm and on the line connecting Yangchi (SJ 4) and the tip of the olecranon, 2 cun proximal to the dorsal crease of the wrist, between the radius and the ulna.

Actions and indications: To clear away Heat, relieve exterior syndrome, activate Blood flow in the channels and collaterals and improve hearing; indicated for common cold, high fever, mumps, pneumonia, headache, facial paralysis, dysfunction of the tempomanidibular joint, tinnitus, deafness, arthritis of the elbow, paralysis of the radial nerve, arthritis of the wrist, finger pain, paralysis due to stroke, sprain of the lumbar muscle, stiff neck and enuresis.

Manipulation: Puncture 0. 5-1 cun perpendicularly. Moxibustion is applicable.

Notes: This is the Luo-Connecting point of the Triple-Jiao Channel of Hand-Shaoyang. It is one of the eight crossing points of the eight extraordinary channels which communicates with the Yangwei Channel.

(22) Zhigou (SJ 6):

Location: On the dorsal side of the forearm and on the line connecting Yangchi (SJ 5) and the olecranon, 3 cun proximal to the dorsal crease of the wrist, between the radius and the ulna.

Actions and indications: To regulate flow of Qi, clear away Heat, lower down the adverse upward flow of Qi and promote bowel movements; indicated for asthma, angina pectoris, intercostal neuralgia, pleuritis, hypogalactia, habitual constipation, aching in the back and shoulder, sprain of the lumbar muscle and aphasia.

Manipulation: Puncture 0. 8-1 cun perpendicularly. Moxibustion is applicable.

Notes: This is the Jing-River point of the Triple-Jiao Channel of Hand-Shaoyang.

(23) Jianliao (SJ 14):

Location: In the shoulder, posterior to Jianyu (LI 15), in the depression inferior and posterior to the acromion when the arm is abducted.

Actions and indications: To relax muscles and tendons, activate flow of Blood in the channels and collaterals, promote Blood flow of channels to expel Wind; indicated for periarthritis of shoulder, hypertension and paralysis due to stroke.

Manipulation: Puncture 1.5 cun perpendicularly or downward obliquely. Moxibustion is applicable.

(24) Shangyang (LI 1):

Location: On the radial side of the distal segment of the index finger, 0.1 cun from the corner of the nail.

Actions and indications: To relieve exterior syndrome, reduce fever, clear away Heat from the Lung and benefit throat; indicated for toothache, laryngitis, pharyngitis, tonsilitis and mumps.

Manipulation: Puncture 0.1 cun or prick to cause bleeding. Moxibustion is applicable.

Notes: This is the Jing-Well point of the Large Intestine Channel of Hand-Yangming.

(25) Erjian (LI 2):

Location: In the depression of the radial side, distal to the 2nd metacarpophalangeal joint when a loose fist is made.

Actions and indications: To clear away Heat from the Lung, benefit the throat, reduce fever and subdue swelling; indicated for toothache, pharyngitis, laryngitis, tonsilitis, epistaxis, stye and periarthritis of shoulder.

Manipulation: Puncture 0.3-0.5 cun perpendicularly. Moxibustion is applicable.

Notes: This is the Ying-Spring point of the Large Intestine Channel of Hand-Yangming.

(26) Sanjian (LI 3):

Location: In the depression of the radial side, posterior to the 2nd metacapophalangeal joint when a loose fist is made.

Actions and indications: To clear away Heat, disperse Wind, promote flow of Qi and regulate the function of the Fu organs; indicated for acute conjunctivitis, glaucoma, toothache, laryngitis, pharyngitis, tonsilitis, enteritis, diarrhea, periarthritis of shoulder and swelling and pain of hand.

Manipulation: Puncture 0.3-0.5 cun perpendicularly. Moxibustion is applicable.

Notes: This is the Shu-Stream point of the Large Intestine Channel of Hand-Yangming.

(27) Hegu (LI 4):

Location: On the dorsum of hand, between the 1st and the 2nd metacarpal bones, and on the radial side of the midpoint of the 2nd metacarpal bone.

Actions and indications: To expel Wind, clear away Heat, promote Blood flow in the channels and collaterals; indicated for common cold, headache, laryngitis, tonsilitis, rhinitis, toothache, deafness, tinnitus, trigeminal neuralgia, spasm of the facial muscles, facial paralysis, neurosis, hysteria, schizophrenia, sprain of the lumbar muscle, hemiplegia of stroke, stiff neck, hiccup, dysmenorrhea, amenorrhea, infantile convulsion, surgical operation on the head and neck as an anaesthesia method.

Manipulation: Puncture 0. 5-0. 8 cun perpendicularly. Moxibustion is applicable. Be sure not to puncture this point in a pregnant woman.

Notes: This is the Yuan-Source point of the Large Intestine Channel of Hand-Yangming.

(28) Pianli (LI 6):

Location: On the radial side of the dorsal surface of the dorearm, and on the line connecting Yangxi (LI 5) and Quchi (LI 11), 3 cun above the crease of the wrist, when the elbow is flexed.

Actions and indications: To regulate flow of the Lung Qi and promote water metabolism; indicated for aching of the arm, laryngitis, tonsilitis, epistaxis, deafness, tinnitus, conjunctivitis and edema.

Manipulation: Puncture 0. 3-0. 5 cun obliquely. Moxibustion is applicable.

Notes: This is the Luo-Connecting point of the Large Intestine Channel of Hand-Yangming.

(29) Quchi (LI 11):

Location: When the elbow is slightly flexed, at the lateral end of the cubital crease, at the midpoint of the line connecting Chize (LU 5) and the external humeral epicondyle.

Actions and indications: To clear away Heat, remove Dampness and benefit movements of the joints; indicated for hemiplegia in stroke, arthritis of the elbow, tennis elbow, sprain of the lumbar muscle, common cold, laryngitis, tonsilitis, toothache, stye, mastitis, anemia, abdominal pain, hypertension, goiter, allergic diseases and dermotological diseases.

Manipulation: Puncture 0. 5-0. 8 cun perpendicularly. Moxibustion is applicable.

Notes: This is the He-Sea point of the Large Intestine Channel of Hand-Yangming.

(30) Jianyu (LI 15):

Location: On the shoulder, superior to the deltoid muscle, in the depression anterior and inferior to the olecranon when the arm is abducted or raised on the level of the shoulder.

Actions and indications: To benefit movement of the joint and disperse Wind and Heat; indicated for hemiplegia in stroke, hypertension, periarthritis, mastitis and urticaria.

Manipulation: Puncture 0. 5-1 cun perpendicularly. Moxibustion is applicable.

4. The acupoints in the lower limbs

(1) Yinbai (SP 1):

Location: In the medial side of the distal segment of the great toe, 0. 1 cun from the corner of the nail.

Actions and indications: To regulate menstruation, relieve bleeding, strengthen the Spleen and restore the depleted yang; indicated for dysfunctional uterine bleeding, hematuria, gastrointestinal bleeding, bleeding gums, epistaxis, acute gastroenteris, coma and infantile convulsion.

Manipulation: Puncture obliquely 0. 1 cun or prick to cause bleeding. Moxibustion is applicable.

Notes: This is the Jing-Well point of the Spleen Channel of Foot-Taiyin.

(2) Gongsun (SP 4):

Location: In the medial border of the foot, anterior and inferior to the proximal end of the 1st metatarsal bone.

Actions and indications: To strengthen the Spleen, remove Dampness, regulate the function of the Middle-Jiao and clear away Heat; indicated for gastritis, gastric ulcer, indigestion, enteritis, dysentery, hepatitits, myocarditis, pleuritis, edema on the head or face and epilepsy.

Manipulation: Puncture 0. 5-1 cun perpendicularly. Moxibustion is applicable.

Notes: This is the Luo-Connecting point of the Spleen Channel of Foot-Taiyin. It is also one of the eight crossing points of the eight extraordinary channels which communicates with the Chong Channel.

(3) Shanqiu (SP 5):

Location: In the depression anterior and inferior to the medial malleolus, at the midpoint of the line connecting the tubersity of the navicular bone and the tip of the medial malleolus.

Actions and indications: To strengthen the Spleen, remove Dampness, regulate the function of the gastrointestine and promote bowel movement; indicated for gastritis, enteritis, diarrhea, indigestion, edema, constipation, diseases of the ankle or its peripheral soft tissues and infantile convulsion.

Manipulation: Puncture 0. 5-0. 8 cun obliquely forwards. Moxibustion is applicable.

Notes: This is the Jing-River point of the Spleen Channel of Foot-Taiyin.

(4) Sanyinjiao (SP 6):

Location: On the medial side of the leg, 3 cun above the tip of the medial malleolus, posterior to the medial border of the tibia.

Actions and indications: To strengthen the Spleen, remove Dampness, regulate the function of the Liver and the Kidney; indicated for enuresis, retention of urine, irregular menstruation, dysfunctional uterine bleeding, erosion of the cervix of uterus, paralysis of the lower limbs, gastritis, enteritis and insomnia.

Manipulation: Puncture 1-1. 5 cun perpendicularly. Moxibustion is applicable.

Notes: This is the crossing point of the Spleen Channel of Foot-

Taiyin, the Kidney Channel of Foot-Shaoyin and the Liver Channel of Foot-Jueyin. According to the ancient literature, it should not be needled in pregnant women.

(5) Diji (SP 8):

Location: On the medial side of the leg, on the line connecting the tip of the medial malleolus and Yinlingquan (SP 9), 3 cun below Yinlingquan (SP 9).

Actions and indications: To strengthen the Spleen, remove Dampness and regulate menstruation and flow of Blood; indicated for gastritis, enteritis, irregular menstruation, dysmenorrhea, dysfunctional uterine bleeding, hysteromyoma, aspermia, mastitis, and paralysis of the lower limbs.

Manipulation: Puncture 1-2 cun perpendicularly. Moxibustion is applicable.

Notes: This is the Xi-Cleft point of the Spleen Channel of Foot-Taiyin.

(6) Yinlingquan (SP 9):

Location: On the medial side of the leg, in the depression posterior and inferior to the medial condyle of the tibia.

Actions and indications: To strengthen the Spleen, induce diuresis, benefit the function of the Lower-Jiao; indicated for enuresis, retention of urine, urinary infection, ascites, enteritis, dysentery, nocturnal emission, impotence, dysmenorrhea, irregular menstruation, arthritis of the knee, and paralysis of the lower limbs.

Manipulation: Puncture 0.5-1 cun perpendicularly. Moxibustion is applicable.

Notes: This is the He-Sea point of the Spleen Channel of Foot-Taiyin.

(7) Xuehai (SP 10):

Location: With the knee flexed, on the medial side of the thigh, 2 cun above the superior medial corner of the patella, on the prominence of the medial head of the quadriceps muscle of the thigh.

Actions and indications: To regulate menstruation and Blood, strengthen the Spleen and induce diuresis; indicated for eczema, urticaria, cutaneous pruritis, neurodermatitis, anemia, irregular menstruation, dysfunctional uterine bleeding, endometritis, testitis, arthritis of the knee, and ulcers in the lower limb.

Manipulation: Puncture 1-1. 5 cun perpendicularly or upward obliquely. Moxibustion is applicable.

(8) Dadun (LR 1):

Location: On the lateral side of the distal segment of the great toe, 0. 1 cun from the corner of the nail.

Actions and indications: To restore the depleted Yang and rescue patient from collapse, regulate menstruation and treat gonorrhea; indicated for cerebrovascular diseases, epilepsy, angina pectoris, hernia, cystitis, prostratitis, gonorrhea, testitis, dysfunctional uterine bleeding, incarcerated inguinal hernia, and paralysis of the lower limbs.

Manipulation: Puncture 0. 1-0. 2 cun obliquely or prick to cause bleeding. Moxibustion is applicable.

Notes: This is the Jing-Well point of the Liver Channel of Foot-Jueyin.

(9) Xingjian (LR 2):

Location: On the insep of the foot, between the 1st and the 2nd toes, at the junction of the red and white skin proximal to the margin of the web.

Actions and indications: To clear away Heat from the Liver, calm the mind, regulate menstruation and consolidate the Chong Channel; indicated for schizophrenia, epilepsy, neurosis, tinnitus, facial paralysis, laryngitis, tonsilitis, epistaxis, angina pectoris, gastritis, enteritis, cystitis, urinary inflammation, enuresis, retention of urine, dysmenorrha, dysfunctional uterine bleeding, arthritis of the knee and inflammation of the metatarsophalangeal joint.

Manipulation: Puncture 0. 5-0. 8 cun perpendicularly. Moxibustion is applicable.

Notes: This is the Ying-Spring point of the Liver Channel of Foot-Jueyin.

(10) Taichong (LR 3):

Location: On the insep of the foot, in the depression of the posterior end of the 1st interosseous metatarsal space.

Actions and indications: To clear away Heat from the Liver, calm endogenous Wind, relieve depression and promote flow of the Liver Qi; indicated for epilepsy, hysteria, neurosis, convulsion, dizziness, headache, supraorbital neuralgia, trigeminal neuralgia, facial paralysis, spasm of the facial muslces, conjunctivitis, optic neuritis, glaucoma, epistaxis, laryngitis, pharyngitis, cervical lymphonoditis, hyperthyroidism, hernia, intercostal neuralgia, lumbo-sacral radiculoneuritis, pain in the lower leg, hepatitis, angina pectoris, spasm of the diaphragm, gastritis, enteritis, cystitis, urinary infection, gonorrhea, testitis, enuresis, dysfunctional uterine bleeding and mastitis.

Manipulation: Puncture 0. 5-1 cun perpendicularly. Moxibustion is applicable.

Notes: This is the Shu-Stream and Yuan-Source points of the Liver Channel of Foot-Jueyin.

(11) Ligou (LR 5):

Location: On the medial side of the lower leg, 5 cun above the tip of the medial malleolus, at the centre of the medial aspect of the femur.

Actions and indications: To soothe flow of the Liver Qi, regulate menstruation and relieve leukorrea; indicated for cystitis, urethritis, testitis, eczema of the scrotum, nocturnal emission, impotence, hypersexualism, retention of urine, hernia with pain, amenorrhea, irregular menstruation, erosion of the uterine cervix, dysfunctional uterine bleeding, inguinal lymphonoditis,.

Manipulation: Puncture 0. 5-0. 8 cun perpendicularly. Moxibustion is applicable.

Notes: This is the Luo-Connecting point of the Liver Channel of Foot-Jueyin.

(12) Ququan (LR 8):

Location: On the medial side of the knee, at the medial end of the popliteal crease when the knee is flexed, posterior to the medial epicondyle of tibia, in the depression of the anterior border of the insertions of semimembranous and semitendinous muscles.

Actions and indications: To tonify the Liver and the Kidney, clear away Heat and remove Dampness; indicated for chronic persisting hepatitis, enteritis, dysentery, nephritis, hernia, prostratitis, nocturnal emission, impotence, retention of urine, irregular menstruation, prolapse of uterus, amenorrhea, sterility, vulvitis, pruritus, and diseases of the knee joint and its surrounding soft tissues.

Manipulation: Puncture 0.6-1.2 cun. Moxibustion is applicable.

Notes: This is the He-Sea point of the Liver Channel of Foot-Jueyin.

(13) Yongquan (KI 1):

Location: In the sole, in the depression occurring on the anterior part of the sole with the foot is in a plantal position, approximately at the junction of the anterior one third and posterior two thirds of the line connecting the base of the 2nd anb 3rd toes and heel.

Actions and indications: To nourish the Kidney-Yin, calm the Liver to suppress endogenous Wind; indicated for headache, dizziness, hypertension, shock, sun-stroke, hoarseness, pharyngitis or laryngitis, acute tonsilitis, palpitation, jaundice, prolaspe of uterus, hemiplegia due to stroke, spasm of muscles in the lower leg, infantile convulsion, thrush, papula, gastrospasm, enuresis, retention of urine, pain in the soles, insomnia, hysteria and schizophrenia.

Manipuation: Puncture 0.5-1 cun. Moxibustion is contraindicated.

Notes: This is the Jing-Well point of the Kidney Channel of Foot-Shaoyin.

(14) Taixi (KI 3):

Location: On the medial aspect of the foot, posterior to the medial malleolus, in the depression between the tip of the medial malleolus and the heel.

Actions and indications: To mourish Yin, supplement Kidney, reinforce the Spleen and support the Lung; indicated for toothache, pharyngitis or laryngitis, tinnitus, bald, emphysema, neurosism, lumbago, paralysis of lower limb, heel pain, and diseases of the urinary system.

Manipulation: Puncture 0.5-1 cun perpendicularly. Moxibustion

is applicable.

Notes: This is the Shu-Stream and Yuan-Source points of the Kidney Channel of Foot-Shaoyin.

(15) Zhaohai (KI 6):

Location: On the medial side of the foot, in the depression below the tip of the medial malleolus.

Actions and indications: To nourish Yin, calm the mind, and regulate defecation and urination; indicated for acute tonsilitis, pharyngitis or laryngitis, rheumatic arthritis, angitis of the lower limbs, epilepsy, hysteria, insomnia, constipation, and diseases of the urinary system and the reproductive system.

Manipulation: Puncture 0. 5-1 cun perpendicularly. Moxibustion is applicable.

Notes: One of the eight crossing points of the eight extraordinary channels which communicates with Yinqiao Channel.

(16) Fuliu (KI 7):

Location: On the medial aspect of the lower leg, 2 cun directly above Taixi (KI 3), anterior to the heel.

Actions and indications: To tonify the Kidney, nourish Yin, induce diuresis and relieve edema; indicated for edema, absence of sweat, night sweat, toothache, lumbago, paralysis of the lower limbs, bleeding of haemorrhoids and diseases of the urinary and the reproductive systems.

Manipulation: Puncture 0. 8-1 cun perpendicularly. Moxibustion is applicable.

Notes: This is the Jing-River point of the Kidney Channel of Foot-Shaoyin.

(17) Jiaoxin (KI 9):

Location: On the medial aspect of the lower leg, 2 cun directly above Taixi (KI 2), 0. 5 cun anterior to Fuliu (KI 7), posterior to the medial border of tibia.

Actions and indications: To tonify the Kidney, regulate menstruation, clear away Heat and induce diuresis; indicated for enteritis, dysentery, constipation and gynecological diseases.

Manipulation: Puncture 0. 6-1 cun perpendicularly. Moxibustion

is applicable.

Notes: This is the Xi-Cleft point of the Yinqiao Channel.

(18) Zhubin (KI 9):

Location: On the medial aspect of the leg and on the line connecting Taixi (KI 3) and Yingu (KI 10), 5 cun above Taixi (KI 3), inferior and medial to the gastrocnemius muscle belly.

Actions and indications: To regulate the function of the Liver and the Kidney, tonify the Kidney and the Liver, clear away Heat and induce diuresis, indicative for schizophrenia, epilepsy, neurogenic vomiting, and systremma.

Manipulation: Puncture 0. 5-0. 8 cun perpendicularly. Moxibustion is applicable.

Notes: This is the Xi-Cleft point of the Yinwei Channel.

(19) Zhiyin (BL 67):

Location: In the lateral side of the distal segment of the little toe, 0. 1 cun from the corner of the nail.

Actions and indications: To dredge channels, promote flow of Blood in the collaterals and clear away Heat from the head; indicative for improper fetal position, dystocia, retained placenta, headache, dizziness, bleeding of bulbar conjunctiva, leukoma, stuffy nose, retention of urine, nocturnal emission, intussusception and paralysis due to stroke.

Manipulation: Puncture 0. 1 cun superficially. Moxibustion is applicable.

Notes: This is the Jing-Well point of the Bladder Channel of Foot-Taiyang.

(20) Shugu (BL 65):

Location: On the lateral side of the foot, posterior to the 5th metatarsophalangeal joint, at the junction of the white and red skin.

Actions and indications: To promote flow of Blood in the channels and collaterals, clear away Heat and dispel Wind; indicative for hypertension, headache, dizziness, tinnitus, deafness, blepharitis ciliaris, dacryostenosis, pain in the back and lumbar region, systremma and various kinds of cutaneous or subcutaneous inflammations.

Manipulation: Puncture 0. 3-0. 5 cun perpendicularly. Moxibus-.

tion is applicable.

Notes: This is the Shu-Stream point of the Bladder Channel of Foot-Taiyang.

(21) Jinmen (KI 63):

Location: In the lateral side of the foot, directly below the anterior border of the external malleolus, on the inferior border of the cuboid bone.

Actions and indications: To activate Blood flow in the channels and collaterals, clear away Heat from the head and tranquilize the mind; indicated for arthritis, sprain of the ankle, hernia and epilepsy.

Manipulation: Puncture 0.3-0.5 cun perpendicularly. Moxibustion is applicable.

(22) Shenmai (KI 62):

Location: In the lateral side of the foot, in the depression directly below the tip of the external malleolus.

Actions and indications: To activate Blood flow in the channels and collaterals, promote flow of Qi, tranquilize the mind and clear away Heat from the head; indicative for paralysis in the lower limbs, arthritis, sprain of the ankle, dizziness, headache, insomnia, stiff neck and diarrhea.

Notes: Puncture 0.3-0.5 cun perpendicularly. Moxibustion is applicable.

Notes: One of the eight crossing points of the eight extraordinary channels, which communicates with the Yangqiao Channel.

(23) Kunlun (KI 60):

Location: Posterior to the external malleolus, in the depression between the tip of the external malleolus and the heel.

Actions and indications: To relax muscles and tendons, clear away Heat from the head and improve eyesight; indicated for sciatica, lumbago, paralysis in the lower limbs, sprain of the ankle, headache, dizziness and epistaxis.

Manipulation: Puncture 0.5-1 cun perpendicularly. Moxibustion is applicable.

Notes: This is the Jing-Well point of the Bladder Channel of

Foot-Taiyang.

(24) Feiyang (BL 58):

Location: On the posterior side of the lower leg, posterior to the external malleolus, 7 cun directly above Kunlun (KI 60) and 1 cun lateral and inferior to Chengshan (KI 57).

Actions and indications: To relax muscles and tendons, activate Blood flow in the collaterals, clear away Heat and subdue swelling; indicated for paralysis in the lower limbs, hemorrhoids and dizziness.

Manipulation: Puncture 1-1. 5 cun perpendicularly. Moxibustion is applicable.

Notes: This is the Luo-Connecting point of the Bladder Channel of Foot-Taiyang.

(25) Chengshan (BL 57):

Location: On the posterior midline of the leg, between Weizhong (BL 40) and Kunlun (BL 60), in a pointed depression formed below the belly of gastrocnemius muscle when the leg is stretched or the heel is lifted.

Actions and indications: To relax muscles and tendons, activate flow of Blood in the collaterals, and regulate the function of the intestine; indicated for gastrospasm, dysmenorrhea, abdominal pain, sciatica, systremma, paralysis of the lower limbs, constipation, hemorrhoids and prolapse of retum.

Manipulation: Puncture 1-2 cun perpendicularly. Moxibustion is applicable.

(26) Weizhong (BL 40):

Location: At the midpoint of the popliteal crease, between the tendons of the biceps muscle of the thigh and semitendinous muscle.

Actions and indications: To clear away Heat, dispel Wind, relax muscles and tendons and activate Blood flow in the collaterals; indicated for sun-stroke, acute gastroenteritis, pain in the back and lumbar region, sciatica, pain of knees, paralysis in the lower limbs, systremma, urticaria, rebulla, psoriasis, boils, enuresis, retention of urine and epistaxis.

Manipulation: Puncture 1-1. 5 cun perpendicularly or prick to cause bleeding. Moxibustion is applicable.

Notes: This is the He-Sea point of the Bladder Channel of Foot-Taiyang.

(27) Weiyang (BL 39):

Location: At the lateral end of the popliteal crease, medial to the tendon of the biceps muscle of the thigh.

Actions and indications: To dredge the water metabolism in the Triple-Jiao, promote Blood flow in the channels and collaterals; indicated for ascites and pain of knees.

Manipulation: Puncture 1-1. 5 cun perpendicularly. Moxibustion is applicable.

Notes: This is the Luo-Connecting point of the Bladder Channel of Foot-Taiyang.

(28) Zhibian (BL 54):

Location: In the gluteal region, at the level of the 4th posterior sacral foramen, 3 cun lateral to the median sacral spine.

Actions and indications: To relax tendons and muscles, activate Blood flow in the collaterals, strengthen the loins and knees; indicated for sequela of cerebrovascular diseases, sciatica, sprain of the lumbar muscle, piriformis syndrome, progressive myodystrophy, cystitis and urethritis.

Manipulation: Puncture 1-1. 5 cun perpendicularly. Moxibustion is applicable.

(29) Zulinqi (GB 41):

Location: On the lateral side of the insep of the foot, posterior to the 4th metatarsophalangeal joint, in the depession lateral to the tendon of extensor muscle of the little toe.

Actions and indications: To soothe the flow of the Liver Qi, relieve mental depression, tranquilize Wind and purge Fire; indicated for headache, dizziness, hemiplegia in stroke, heel pain, intermittent fever, dyspnea, irregular menstruation, improper fetal position, and mastitis,

Manipulation: Puncture 0. 3-0. 5 cun perpendicularly. Moxibustion is applicable.

Notes: This is the Shu-Stream point of the Gallbladder Channel of Foot-Shaoyang. It is also one of the eight crossing points of the eight extraordinary channels, which communicates with the Dai Channel.

(30) Xuanzhong (GB 39):

Location: In the lateral side of the leg, 3 cun above the tip of the external malleolus, on the anterior border of the fibula.

Actions and indications: To promote Blood flow in the channels, activate collaterals, strengthen the tendons and bones; indicated for sequela of the cerebrovascular diseases, diseases of the ankle and its surrounding soft tissues, myelitis, sprain of the lumbar muscle, stiff neck, headache, tonsilitis, rhinitis, and epistaxis.

Manipulation: Puncture 1-1.5 cun perpendicularly. Moxibustion is applicable.

Notes: This is one of the eight confluential points where marrow converges.

(31) Guangming (GB 37):

Location: In the lateral side of the leg, 5 cun above the tip of the external malleolus, on the anterior border of the fibula.

Actions and indications: To soothe flow of the Liver Qi, improve eyesight, promote Blood flow in the channels and activate collaterals; indicated for blepharitis ciliaris, night blindness, ametropia, arthritis of the knee, and sprain of the lumbar muscle.

Manipulation: Puncture 1-1.5 cun perpendicularly. Moxibustion is applicable.

Notes: This is the Luo-Connecting point of the Gallbladder Channel of Foot-Shaoyang.

(32) Yanglingquan (GB 34):

Location: In the lateral side of the leg, in the depression inferior and anterior to the head of the fibula.

Actions and indications: To soothe flow of the Liver Qi, benefit the Gallbladder, strengthen the loins and knees; indicated for arthritis of the knee and diseases of its surrounding soft tissues, paralysis of the lower limbs, sprain of the ankle, periarthritis of the shoulder, stiff neck, intercostal neuralgia, sprain of the lumbar muscle, pain of the arm muscles after injection, hypertension, hepatitis, cholecystitis, cholelithiasis, colic of the gallbladder, biliary ascariasis and habitual constipation.

Manipulation: Puncture 1-1. 5 cun perpendicularly. Moxibustion is applicable.

Notes: This is the He-Sea point of the Gallbladder Channel of Foot-Shaoyang. It is also one of the eight confluential points where the tendons converge.

(33) Huantiao (GB 30):

Location: On the lateral side of the thigh, at the junction of the middle third and lateral third of the line connecting the prominence of the great trochanter and the sacral hiatus when the patient is in a lateral recumbent position with the thigh flexed.

Actions and indications: To promote Blood flow in the channels, activate collaterals, expel Wind and disperse Cold; indicative for diseases of the hip joint and its surrounding soft tissues, sciatica, lumbago, paralysis of stroke, swelling and pain of knees or ankles, and rubella.

Manipulation: Puncture 2-3. 5 cun perpendicularly or slightly toward the spine. Moxibustion is applicable.

Notes: This is the crossing point of the Gallbladder Channel of Foot-Shaoyang and the Bladder Channel of Foot-Taiyang.

(34) Lidui (ST 45):

Location: In the lateral side of the distal segment of the 2nd toe, 0. 1 cun from the corner of the nail.

Actions and indications: To restore consciousness, regulate the function of the Stomach and regulate flow of Qi; indicative for shock, collapse, sleepiness, epilepsy, hysteria, facial paralysis, epistaxis, rhinitis, toothache, tonsilitis, laryngitis, gastritis, hepatitis, indigestion and paralysis in the lower limbs.

Manipulation: Puncture 0. 1 cun superficially. Moxibustion is applicable.

Notes: This is the Jing-Well point of the Stomach Channel of Foot-Yangming.

(35) Neiting (ST 44):

Location: In the insep of the foot, between 2nd and the 3rd toes, at the junction of the white and the red skin proximal to the margin of the web.

Actions and indications: To regulate the function of the Stomach, strengthen the Spleen, clear away Heat from the Heart and tranquilize the mind; indicated for gastritis, gastrospasm, spasm of diaphragm, enteritis, dysentery, common cold, headache, facial paralysis, epistaxis, spasm of the vocal fold, tinnitus, conjunctivitis, toothache, urticaria, dysmenorrhea and hysteria.

Manipulation: Puncture 0. 3-0. 5 cun perpendicularly. Moxibustion is applicable.

Notes: This is the Ying-Spring point of the Stomach Channel of Foot-Yangming.

(36) Chongyang (ST 42):

Location: At the highest point of the insep of the foot, between the tendons of the long extensor muscle of the great toe and long extensor muscle of toes, where the pulsation of the dorsal artery of foot is palpable.

Actions and indications: To regulate the function of the Stomach, dissolve Dampness, tranquilize the mind and promote Blood flow in the collaterals, indicative for toothache, facial paralysis, gastritis, indigestion, dizziness, rheumatic arthritis and sprain of the foot.

Manipulation: Puncture 0. 2-0. 5 cun perpendicularly. Moxibustion is applicable.

Notes: This is the Yuan-Source point of the Stomach Channel of Foot-Yangming.

(37) Fenglong (ST 40):

Location: In the anterior and lateral side of the leg, 8 cun above the tip of the external malleolus, lateral to Tiaokou (ST 38) and two finger breadth from the anterior crest of tibia.

Actions and indications: To regulate the function of the Stomach, strengthen the Spleen, dissolve Phlegm and remove Dampness, indicative for bronchitis, bronchial asthma, injury of the soft tissues in the chest, gastritis, peptic ulcers, neurogenic vomiting, enteritis, hypertension, hyperlipemia, sequela of the cerebrovascular diseases, auditary vertigo, hysteria, schizophrenia, encephalitis B, obesity, nephritis, cystitis, urethritis, amenorrhea and dysfunctional uterine bleeding.

Manipulation: Puncture 1-1.5 cun perpendicularly. Moxibustion is applicable.

Notes: This is the Luo-Connecting point of the Stomach Channel of Foot-Yangming.

(38) Xiajuxu (ST 39):

Location: In the anterior and lateral side of the leg, 9 cun below Dubi (ST 35) and one finger breadth (middle finger) from the anterior crest of tibia.

Actions and indications: To clear away Heat, remove Dampness, tranquilize the mind and relieve convulsion, indicative for gastritis, enteritis, intercostal neuralgia, mastitis, rheumatic arthritis, paralysis in the lower limbs, epilepsy and schizophrenia.

Manipulation: Puncture 1-1.5 cun perpendicularly. Moxibustion is applicable.

Notes: This is the lower-Sea point of the Small Intestine Channel of Hand-Taiyang.

(39) Shangjuxu (ST 37):

Location: In the anterolateral side of the leg, 6 cun below Dubi (ST 35), one finger breadth (middle finger) from the crest of tibia.

Actions and indications: To regulate the function of the Stomach, strengthen the Spleen, dredge flow of Blood in the channels and regulate flow of Qi; indicated for gastritis, peptic ulcers, enteritis, intestinal obstruction, appendicitis, indigestion, hepatitis, nephritis, arthritis and paralysis of the lower limbs.

Manipulation: Puncture 1-1.5 cun perpendicularly. Moxibustion is applicable.

Notes: This is the lower-Sea point of the Large Intestine Channel of Hand-Yangming.

(40) Zusanli (ST 36):

Location: In the anterolateral side of the leg, 3 cun below Dubi (ST 35), one finger breadth (middle finger) from the crest of tibia.

Actions and indications: To promote flow of Blood in the channels and collaterals, regulate Qi and Blood, normalize the function of the

85

Stomach, strengthen the Spleen, support the Vital Qi and supplement the primordial Qi, indicative for such diseases of the digestive system as gastritis, gastrospasm, peptic ulcers, gastroptosis, enteritis, dysentery, appendicitis, intestinal obstruction, hepatitis, ascariasis, indigestion, infantile anorexia and aiding in gastrofibroscopy; such diseases of the circulatory system as hypertension, hyperlipemia, coronary heart disease, angina pectoris and rheumatism; such diseases of the respiratory system as bronchitis and bronchial asthma; such diseases of the urinary and reproductive systems such as nephritis, renal colic, cystitis, enuresis, impotence, irregular menstruation, dysfunctional uterine bleeding and pelvic inflammation; and such miscellaneous diseases as dysfunction of the tempomandibular joint, facial paralysis, myopia, hyperopia, tinnitus, deafness, morning sickness, mastitis, urticaria, rheumatoid arthritis, shock and insomnia.

Manipulation: Puncture 0.5-1 cun perpendicularly. Moxibustion is applicable.

Notes: This is the He-Sea point of the Stomach Channel of Foot-Yangming. It is also an important point for health care because it has a strong effect of enhancing the constitution.

(41) Liangqiu (ST 34):

Location: With the knee flexed, on the anterior side of the thigh and on the line connecting the anterosuperior illiac spine and the superiolateral corner of patella, 2 cun above this corner.

Actions and indications: To relax muscles and tendons, activate collaterals, subdue swelling and relieve pain; indicated for rheumatic arthritis, suprapetallar bursitis, chondromalacia patellae, mastitis, acute gastritis, enteritis, and dysmenorrhea.

Manipulation: Puncture 0.5-1 cun perpendicularly. Moxibustion is applicable.

Notes: This is the Xi-Cleft point of the Stomach Channel of Foot-Yangming.

Commonly Used Extra Points

Yintang (EX-HN3):

Location: On the forehead, at the midpoint between the bilateral eyebrows.

Actions and indications: To clear away Heat, expel Wind, relieve convulsion and arrest pain; indicated for headache, acute conjunctivitis, trigeminal pain and facial paralysis.

Manipulation: Puncture 0. 3-0. 4 cun perpendicularly or subcutaneously or prick to cause bleeding.

Shixuan (EX-UE11):

Location: At the tips of the ten fingers, 0. 1 cun from the corners of the nails.

Actions and indications: To purge Heat, restore consciousness, and relieve convulsion; indicated for shock, coma, high fever, sunstroke, epilepsy, hysteria, infantile convulsion and numbness of the fingers.

Manipulation: Puncture 0. 1-0. 2 cun superficially, or prick to cause bleeding.

Sifeng (EX-UE10):

Location: Four points on one hand, on the palmar side of the 2nd and 5th fingers, and at the center of the proximal interphalangeal joints.

Actions and indications: To relieve malnutrition, eliminate retained food, dissolve Phlegm and induce bowel movement; indicated for whooping cough, arthritis of the fingers and intestinal ascariasis.

Manipulation: Prick with three edged needle to press out yellow-white transparent fluid.

Baxie (EX-UE9):

Location: Four points on the dorsum of each hand, at the junction of the white and red skin proximal to the margin of the web between each two of the five fingers of one hand.

Actions and indications: To expel pathogen, activate collaterals, clear away Heat and remove toxic substances; indicative for diseases of the fingers, headache, sore throat and bite by snake.

Manipulation: Puncture 0. 3-0. 5 cun obliquely, or prick to cause bleeding. Moxibustion is applicable.

Xiyan (EX-LE5):

Location: With the knee flexed, in the depressions on the both sides of the petallar ligament. The medial and the external points are named Internsl Xiyan and External Xiyan respectively.

Actions and indications: To remove Dampness, activate collaterals, and benefit the movements of the joints; indicated for arthritis of the knee.

Manipulation: Puncture 0. 5-1 cun obliquely, or puncture through the point to the opposite point. Moxibustion is applicable.

Dannang (EX-LE 6):

Location: In the upper part of the medial side of the leg, 2 cun below the depression inferior and anterior to the head of fibula (Yanglingquan, BL 34).

Actions and indications: To clear away Heat, benefit the Gall-bladder, activate collaterals and relieve pain; indicative for acute and chronic cholecystitis, cholelithiasis, biliary tract ascariasis and paralysis of the lower limbs.

Manipulation: Puncture 0. 6-0. 8 cun perpendicularly. Moxibustion is applicable.

Lanweixue (EX-LE 7):

Location: In the upper part of the anterior surface of the leg, 5 cun below Dubi (ST 35), one finger breadth (middle finger) lateral to the anterior border of the tibia.

Actions and indications: To clear away Heat, eliminate pathogen, promote downward flow of Qi in the intestine; indicative for acute or chronic appendicitis, gastritis, indigestion and paralysis of the lower limbs.

Manipulation: Puncture 1-1. 2 cun perpendicularly. Moxibustion is applicable.

Bafeng (EX-LE 10):

Location: Eight points on the inseps of the both feet, at the junction of the red and white skin proximal to the margin of the webs between each two neighboring toes.

Actions and indications: To expel Wind, activate collaterals, clear away Heat and remove toxic substance; indicated for sprain of the feet, hemiplegia due to stroke, and irregular menstruation.

Manipulation: Puncture 0. 1-0. 3 cun perpendicularly. Moxibustion is applicable.

Dingchuan (EX-B 1):

Location: On the back, below the spinous process of the 7th cervical vertebra, 0. 5 cun lateral to the posterior midline.

Actions and indications: To relieve asthma, alleviate cough, facilitate flow of the Lung Qi; indicated for stiff neck, bronchial asthma, bronchitis and urticaria.

Manipulation: Puncture 0. 5-0. 8 cun perpendicularly. Moxibustion is applicable.

Jiaji (EX-B 2):

Location: On the back and lower back, 17 points on each side, below the spinous processes from the 1st thoracic to 5th lumbar vertebrae, 0. 5 cun lateral to the posterior midline.

Actions and indications: To regulate the function of the Zang-Fu organs, and benefit the movements of joint; indicated for sequela of cerebraovascular diseases, spondylitis, syringomyelia, bronchitis, bronchial asthma, neurosism and all the chronic diseases.

Manipulation: Puncture 0. 5-1 cun perpendicularly for the points on the chest, 1-1. 5 cun perpendicularly for the points on the lumbar region. Moxibustion is applicable.

Yaoyan (EX-B 7):

Location: On the lumbar region, below the spinous process of the 4th lumbar vertebra, in the depression 3. 5 cun lateral to the posterior midline.

Actions and indications: To strengthen the loins and tonify the Kidney; indicated for sprain of the lumbar muscle, nephritis, irregular menstruation and testitis.

Manipulation: Puncture 1-1. 5 cun perpendicularly. Moxibustion

is applicable.

Yaoqi (EX-B 9):

Location: In the lower back, 2 cun directly above the tip of the coccyx, in the depression below the sacral horn.

Actions and indications: To tranquilize mind, relieve epilepsy, suppress Wind and dissolve Phlegm; indicated for epilepsy, headache, insomnia and constipation.

Manipulation: Puncture 1. 5-2 cun upward subcutaneously. Moxibustion is applicable.

The Acupuncture-
Moxibustion
Methodology

This is a subject dealing with the concrete methods, manipulating techniques and the mechanism of the methods and
techniques in prevention and treatment of disease with
acupuncture-moxibustion. It includes the needling method, the
moxibusting method, and other methods developed based on these
two major methods. All these methods have different characteristics, but they all give their play by acting on the acupoints and channels and collaterals through which to regulate the functional states
of the human body and to prevent and treat disease.

A General Introduction of Acupuncture-
Moxibustion Methodology

1. Preparation before acupuncture-moxibustion treat-
ment

(1) Selection of the tools for acupuncture: Filiform needle is one

91

of the nine kinds of needles for acupuncture in the ancient times. The filiform needle used today, which is mostly made up of the stainless steel, is constituted by five parts: the tip, the body, the root, the handle and the end. The tip of needle refers to the anterior sharp part of the needle; the main part of the needle between the tip and the handle is known as the body of the needle; the junction of the body of the needle and the handle of the needle is called the root of the needle; the part tangled with metal silk for the convenience of holding the needle is termed the handle of the needle; and the distal part of the handle is referred to as the end of the body.

Careful examination must be performed before using a needle. The needle tip should be round but not blunt, like a pine needle. The needle body must be straight, smooth, hard and elastic, and that with rust or being flexed should not be slected. The root of the needle is not allowed to be rusted or loosened, otherwise it may cause the needle to break. Besides, the needles of different length and different thickness should be chosen in accordance with the different sexes, ages, physiques and constitutions of different patients as well as the depth and the thickness of the area to be needled.

(2) Materials for moxibustion: Mugwort floss made from Chinese mugwort leaves is the main material for moxibustion, which is prepared by drying the leaves first, then grinding them into fine powder and removing the impurity within the powder. It is aromatic in odour and very flammable, and has the functions of promoting Blood flow in the channels and collaterals, warming up the meridians to disperse Cold, restoring the depleted Yang and rescuing patients from collapse. In the past thousands of years, it has been adopted as the main material for moxibustion in the clinic. In addition, rush pith and white mustard seed may also be used as the materials.

(3) Selection of positions: An appropriate patient's position is very important for localization of the acupoints, manipulation of needles, placement of the moxa cone and performance of the moxibustion treatment. The commonly adopted positions in the clinic are as follows.

① Lying position: A supine position is suitable for treatment on the acupoints on the head, face, chest, abdomen, the medial aspects of the arms and legs as well as these on the hands and feet. Patient should lie on his one side when the acupoints on the occipital region, the nape and the back are to be treated. When the acupoints on the occipital region, the nape, the back, the lower back, the gluteal region and the posterior aspects of the legs are to be used, patient should take a prone position. Lying position should be taken for patients who receive acupuncture treatment for the first time, feels nervous, with a weak constitution due to aging or with severe disease, to avoid fainting during acupuncture.

② Sitting position: A supine sitting position should be taken when the acupoints on the forehead, the face, the neck and the upper chest are to be treated. A prone sitting position is suitable for treatment of the acupoints on the vertex, occipital region, the nape, the shoulder and the back. And, a side prone sitting position is applicable for acupoints on the side of the head, the cheeks and the retroauricular region or the acupoints in front of the ear.

(4) Sterilization: This includes disinfection of the instruments, the doctor's fingers and the areas to be treated.

① Sterilization of instruments: There are many methods to sterilize the instruments, but the high pressure sterilization is the one mostly suggested, which is carried out by putting such wrapped tools of acupuncture as the filiform needles into an autoclave and keep them in the autoclave for more than 30 minutes with a pressure of 1. 0-1. 4 kg/cm^3 and a temperature of 115℃-123 ℃. The tools may also be sterilized by being soaked for 30-60 minutes in 75% alcohol solution and used after being dried with a clothing. Besides, they may also be inmmersed in a 0. 1% solution of bromogeramine for 1-2 hours for the purpose of disinfection.

② Sterilization of the doctor's fingers: Before treatment, doctor should clean his fingers thoroughly with soap water or with the cotton-ball immersed in alcohol.

③ Sterilization of the areas to be treated: The skin where the acupoints to be treated are may be sterilized with a cotton ball immersed in 75% alcohol, or with iodine first, then with the alcohol.

The sterilized region must be kept in clean to prevent it from being polluted again.

2. Management of the abnormal condition during acupuncture

(1) Faint during acupuncture: Faint during acupuncture arises from improper body position, emotional stress, general weakness or exertion of strong manipulations during acupuncture, which is clinically manifested as sudden pale, dizziness, vertigo, palpitation, shortness of breath, nausea with a desire to vomit, decrease of the blood pressure, cold limbs, fine, feeble and rapid or deep and fine pulse, or even sudden collapse with coma and incontinence of defecation and urination. When faint occurs, doctor should withdraw the needles at once, advice the patient to lie flat with his head being a little lower than his body, loosen his clothes and keep him warm. Patient with a mild faint may recover a while after drinking some warm boiled water, and most patients with severe faint may recover some time after needling Shuigou (DU 26), Neiguan and Yongquan followed by moxibusting Baihui and Qihai (RN 6). If ne... other measures for first aid should be taken.

(2) Sticking of needle: Sticking of needle refers to an ... condition occurring in manipulating the needle, which ... marked by a feeling of unsmoothness or difficulty in rotating, twisting, lifting, inserting or withdrawing the needles. This condition should be managed differently in accordance with different reasons. If it is caused by emotional stress or spasm of the muscles in the treated area, it may be relieved by retaining the needle for a time longer than normal, pressing the adjacent tissues, or inserting another needle in the adjacent area to alleviate the spasm of muscles. If it is caused by excessive twisting toward one direction, the needle may be withdrawn by rotating the needle toward the opposite direction first and then lifted and inserted gently. And, if it is caused by changes of the body position, the body position must be corrected first.

(3) Bending of the needle: If a doctor is not skilled at inserting the needle and thus exert excessive force, or, if the tip of the needle touches hard tissues, the patient changes his position after insertion

of the needle, the handle of the needle is striked by extra force, or the sticking of needle is not managed properly, bending of needle will occur. If the bending of the needle is not severe, the needle may be withdrawn without any manipulations performed. If the bending angle is very great, the needle may be withdrawn along the direction of the bending. And, if the bending of needle is caused by changes of body position, the body position should be corrected first, then withdraw the needle.

(4) Breaking of needle: Breaking of needle may follow when the needle is strongly rotated, twisted, lifted or inserted, patient changes his position, needles of bad quality are applied, or sticking or bending of needle is not managed promptly. At this time, doctor must keep a silent attitude and ask patient to keep his original position to prevent the broken part of the needle from entering the depth. If a part of the broken needle is still exposed above the skin, the resident part of the needle may be taken out with a forceps. If the needle body has entered the depth, it should be taken out by surgical operations in accordance with its location.

(5) Hematoma: Small ecchymosis due to mild subcutaneous bleeding after withdrawing the needle may subside itself and thus requires no management. Severe swelling and pain with a purplish colour or failure of the patient to move freely due to the swelling and pain should be treated by applying cold compress first to stop bleeding, then the hot compression, or by pressing and kneading the local area mildly to promote dissipation and absorption of the coagulated Blood.

(6) Pneumatothorax: While needling the acupoints in the supraclavicular fossa, the upper border of the sternal notch, the bilateral sides of the 11th thoracic vertebra, and the points above the 8th intercostal space on the line passing through the center of the axillary fossa or the 6th intercostal space on the midclavicular line, traumatic pneumatothorax often occurs as a result of the pleura or the lung being injured by the needle that is inserted in an incorrect direction, angle and depth, which is marked by sudden chest stuffiness, chest pain, shortness of breath or even such manifestations of shock as

dyspnea, cyanosis, perspiration and decrease of the blood pressure. On physical examination, there is widening of the intercostal space, hyperresonant percussion note, dimunition or disappearance of the vescicular breath sounds in the affected side, or even shifting of the tracha to the healthy side. X-ray examination may help to ascertain the diagnosis. Once pneumatothorax occurs, patient should take a semilying position to rest. The mild cases may be treated respectively in accordance with the symptoms. For example, patients with cough may be treated by giving antitussives and antibiotics. For severe cases, however, first aid measures should be adopted, such as extraction of gas by pneumothorax puncture, oxygen inhalation or anti-shock measures.

3. Contraindications of acupuncture-moxibustion

(1) Contraindicated areas: Acupuncture should not be applied or should be applied carefully to the brain, the spinal column, the internal organs, the great vessels and the cutaneous area with infection, ulcer, scar or tumours. Important joints should also be punctured carefully. Besides, moxibustion cannot be applied directly to the five sensory organs on the face, the external genitalia and where the great vessels are, and the lower abdomen and the lumbar and the sacral regions of a woman in menstruation or in pregnancy should not be punctured or should be punctured with great care.

(2) Contraindicated diseases: When patient is in a low functional state as a result of severe dehydration or loss of blood, or has a pulse not identical with his or her symptoms, simultaneously bleeding or persistant bleeding after traumatic injury, acupuncture is not suggested. For cases with Excessive Heat syndrome or fever due to Yin Deficiency, moxibustion is not recommendable.

(3) Contraindicated body conditions: Acupuncture should not be performed at once to patients in severe hungry or fatigue with emotional stress. The manipulation of the needle should not be strong for cases with general weakness.

Acupuncture with Filiform Needle

Filiform needle is the most widely applied needle in the clinic. Its manipulations, thus, serve as a most basic technique that must be mastered in acupuncture treatment.

1. Method of inserting the needle

While inserting the needle, the two hands should be well coordinated. The commonly used methods to insert the needle are as follows:

(1) Nail pressing method: This is a method to insert the needle by holding and inserting the needle with the right hand along the nails of the fingers of the left hand, with the nail of the thumb or the nails of the index finger and the middle finger of the left hand pressing on the acupoint, suitable for insertion of the short needle.

(2) Holding and inserting method: With the thumb and the index finger of the left hand holding a sterilized dry contton ball to fix the tip of the needle at the skin surface where the point to be needled is, rotate the needle with the other hand to insert the needle. This method is called holding and inserting method, which is mainly adopted to insert a long needle.

(3) Spreading and inserting method: This is a method of inserting the needle by spreading the skin of the local area with the thumb and the index finger of the left hand from where the point is located to its sides to tighten the skin first, then insert the needle with the right hand through between the thumb and the index finger of the left hand. It is a method used for the area where the skin is loose.

(4) Lifting-kneading insertion method: With the skin where the point to be treated is picked up by the thumb and the index finger of the left hand, insert the needle with the right hand from the upper part of the skin. This is called the lifting-kneading insertion method, which is mainly applied to acupoints located in the area where the skin and muscle are thin.

2. The angle and depth of needling

In acupuncture treatment, the angle and the depth of needling must be well mastered, because it is a very important link in achieving feeling of Qi, improving therapeutic effects and preventing occurrence of accidents.

The angle of needling refers to the angle formed by the needle and the skin in inserting the needle, according to which the acupuncture can be classified as three kinds: The perpendicular puncture, the oblique puncture and the horizontal puncture. The perpendicular puncture means to insert the needle at an angle of 90° or so with the skin surface, which is applicable to most of the acupoints of the body; the oblique puncture indicates to insert the needle at an angle of 45° or so with the skin surface, which is applicable to the acupoints that cannot be punctured deeply; and the horizontal puncture means to insert the needle at an angle of 15°-20° or so with the skin surface, which is applicable to the acupoints located in the area with thin skin and muscles or used in the case of point to point puncture being adopted.

The depth of needling refers to the depth of the needle body being inserted into the acupoints, which varies with the different diseases conditions and the different positions, as well as the different constitutions and the different body forms of patients which determine the response of the human body to the puncture. The depth of needling must be determined based on a complete consideration of the different disease, location of disease and the different conditions of patients, in order to achieve a better therapeutic effect.

3. The basic manipulations and the supplementary manipulations

To apply manipulations after insertion of the needles is called manipulations of the needles, which is usually classfied as the basic manipulations and the supplementary manipulations.

The basic manipulations include two kinds: The lifting and inserting, and roating and twisting. The former is a manipulation to make the needle do up-down movements within the points when the tip of the needle is inserted to certain depth. Inserting means to insert the needle from the shallow part to the deep part; while lifting means to withdraw the needle from the deep part to the shallow part. The latter is a manipulation to make the needle move back and forth within the point with the thumb, the index finger and the middle finger of the right hand holding the handle of the needle when the tip of the needle is inserted to certain depth. The above two basic manipulations may be adopted alone or jointly, depending on patients' different conditions.

The supplementary manipulations refer to the manipulations aiding in moving the needles in acupuncture treatment. They include pressing, flicking, scraping, shaking, flying, etc. The pressing refers to press or push gently the areas around the acupoint that is needled or the areas along the distribution of the channels where the point is located, which can promote flow of Qi in the channel and help achieve feeling of Qi; the flicking means to flick the handle of the needle gently to make the needle vibrate slightly when the needle is inserted to a certain depth, with an aim to strengthen the feeling of the needling; the scraping indicates to scrape the handle of the needle from its lower part to its upper part with the nails of the thumb, the index finger and the middle finger, which can strengthen the feeling of needling and help spread the feeling; the shaking means to shake the needle body gently by holding the handle of the needle to promote flow of Qi or make the feeling of needle spread toward certain direction; and the flying means to do large scale of twisting and rotating through the thumb and the index finger first when the needle is inserted to certain depth followed by loosing the hand, taking an appearance of a bird with its wings spread, which can strengthen the feeling of needling.

4. Needle transmission and gaining of Qi

Needle transmission refers to various kinds of manipulations employed to help to achieve feeling of Qi, regulate feeling of needling or perform the reinforcement and reducement, following needle insertion. Gaining of Qi, also known as feeling of Qi, means the response of Qi of channel to the stimuli produced by needling. When it occurs, patient will have a soreness, numbness, distension or heaviness sensation in the area around the tip which may spread to a certain direction, while the doctor may experience a moderate or a heavy and tense feeling around the tip of the needle.

Better therapeutic effects can be obtained only when a feeling of Qi occurs and proper reinforcing and reducing manipulations are performed in acupuncture treatment. The influential factors of gaining of Qi are various, mainly involving the constitutions of patients, severity of the diseases and the method of locating the points as well as the manipulations exerted. Generally, patient with flourishing of Qi of channel achieves the feeling of Qi quickly; while one with less Qi of channel achieves the feeling of Qi slowly or cannot achieve the feeling of Qi. When the point is correctly located, the feeling of Qi is easy to obtain; while if the point is not located correctly, feeling of Qi is not easy to achieve. Employment of proper manipulations such as pressing and flicking can irritate the Qi of channel and promote gaining of feeling of Qi.

5. The reinforcing and reducing methods in acupuncture treatment

The manipulations of needles are the main means to produce the reinforcing or reducing effects and to promote the transformation of the intrinsic factors within the body. The commonly used are introduced as follows:

(1) Reinforcing and reducing method by twisting and rotating the needle: When the feeling of Qi is gained, a reinforcing effect may be realized by rotating and twisting the needle at a small angle, with less strength, in a low frequency and in a short time; while a reducing effect may be obtained by rotating and twisting the needle at a great angle, with more strength, in a high frequency and in a longer time.

(2) Reinforcing and reducing method by lifting and inserting the needle: When the feeling of Qi is gained, that lift and insert the needle from the shallow part to the deep part, with more strength exerted while inserting and less strength while lifting, at a small scale, in a low frequency and for a shorter time will produce a reinforcing effect, while a reducing effect will be produced if the needle is lifted and inserted from the deep part to the shallow part, with

100

more strength exerted while lifting and less strength exerted while inserting, in a large scale, in a high frequency and for a longer time.

(3) Reinforcing and reducing method by manipulating the needle rapidly or slowly: When the needle is inserted slowly with less rotating and twisting manipulations applied and quick withdrawal of the needle, it is a method to reinforce; while if the needle is inserted quickly with more roatating and twisting manipulations adopted and slow withdrawal of the needle, it is a method to reduce.

(4) Reinforcing or reducing method by inserting the needle along or against flow of Qi of channel: If the needle is inserted with the tip of the needle directing at the direction of the distribution of the channel, it will cause a reinforcing effect, while if the needle is inserted with the tip against the direction of the distribution of the channel, it will produce a reducing effect.

(5) Reinforcing and reducing method with respiration: Inserting the needle while patient inhales and withdraw the needle while patient exhales will give rise to a reinforcing effect; and inserting the needle while patient exhales and withdraw the needle while patient inhales will cause a reducing effect.

(6) Reinforcing and reducing method by opening and closing the holes: When the needle is withdrawn, that press the hole quickly will cause a reinforcing effect; and enlarging the hole by shaking the needle while withdrawing the needle will produce a reducing effect.

(7) Uniform reinforcing and reducing methods: Following gaining of Qi after insertion, withdrawing the needles after even rotating, twisting, lifting and inserting manipulations are done will cause a uniform reinforcing and reducing effects.

Besides, there are still some compound manipulations which are introduced as follows:

(8) Heat-producing needling: When the needle is inserted into the upper third (the Heaven part) of the normal depth of an acupoint and the feeling of gaining Qi is obtained, rotate and twist the needle with reinforcing method. Then insert the needle deeper to the middle third (the Man part) of the normal depth, and when the feeling of Qi is gained, resume the rotating and twisting reinforcing method

again. After that, insert the needle further to the lower third (the Earth part) to repeat the twisting and rotating manipulation with reinforcing method. Then lift the needle to the upper third slowly. After these procedures are repeated three times, retain the needle in the Earth part tightly. During this process, the reinforcing method by needling with respiration may be adopted in combination. This kind of needling is known as heat-producing needling, which is mostly applied to treatment of arthralgia of Cold type, severe numbness, diseases of the Deficiency-Cold nature, etc.

(9) Cold-producing needling: When the needle is inserted to the lower third of the normal depth of an acupoint and a feeling of Qi is obtained, rotate and twist the needle with reducing method. Then withdraw the needle to the middle third tightly, twist and rotate the needle again with reducing method. After that, withdraw the needle further to the upper third and when feeling of Qi is gained, manipulate the needle with the same method. Then, press the needle slowly to the lower third. Repeat this process three times, and then lift the needle to the upper third to retain there. In this process, the reducing method in reinforcing and reducing manipulations with respiration may be adopted jointly. This kind of method is called cold-producing needling, which is applicable to diseases of an Excess Heat nature such as arthralgia of Heat type, acute carbuncles or furuncles.

6. Retaining and withdrawing of needle

Retaining of needle implies that the needle is retained within the acupoint for some time when the needle is inserted into the acupoint and proper manipulations of needling are applied, with an aim to strengthen the therapeutic effects and for the convenience of continuing the manipulations of needles. The needle may be retained for 20-30 minutes in treatment of most diseases, but it may be retained a longer time with intermittent application of different manipulations during the retaining in the treatment of some special diseases, to keep the stimili at a certain level to enhance the therapeutic effect. In the case of no feeling of Qi being gained, retaining of needle can induce production of the feeling of gaining Qi.

The needle may be withdrawn when the needle is properly manipulated or retained. When withdrawing a needle, the doctor should press the skin around the acupoint with the thumb and the index finger of his left hand first, then rotate and twist the needle gently with his right hand, and lift the needle to subcutaneous region. After that, withdraw the needle quickly out of the skin, and press the hole of needling with a sterilized dry cotton ball to prevent bleeding.

Moxibustion Methods

This is an external therapy by applying a burning or hot mugwort floss or other materials on the acupoint to prevent or treat disease and keep fit through introducing the heat and the effects of the drugs into the human body by the aid of the acupoint and channel. There are many moxibustion methods, the following is only an introduction to the moxibustion with moxa cone, the moxibustion with moxa roll and the moxibustion for keeping health.

1. Moxibustion with a moxa cone

This is of two kinds, the direct moxibustion and the indirect moxibustion. The moxa cone is made from the twisted mugwort floss, taking a shape of cone of varying sizes like that of a wheat seed, lotus seed or half an olive ball. When a cone is completely burnt in moxibustion treatment, it is called one *Zhuang*.

(1) The direct moxibustion: This means to apply the moxa cone directly on the skin to carry out the moxibustion treatment. It can be classfied as the moxibustion without scar and that with scar, depending on the degree of scorching of the skin. The former is performed by applying some vasline in the local skin first, then placing the moxa cone on the vasline and lighting the cone. When 2/5 or 1/4 of the cone is left and patient feels a burning pain in the treated area, change the cone and continue the treatment until the skin in the treated area becomes red without formation of blister. Usually, no scar occurs after the treatment. This method is mainly adopted to

treat diseases of Cold-Deficiency in nature. The latter is performed by applying some garlic juice to the skin first, then placing the moxa cone on the juice and lighting the cone. Each cone must be fully burnt and their ash removed before another cone is placed. Usually there is blister formation after the treatment which will produce diabrosis in 7 days or so and become the ulcer of moxibustion. The ulcer will heal itself within 5-6 weeks, leaving the scar. This method is mainly used to treat such diseases as lung tuberculosis and bronchitis.

(2) Indirect moxibustion: This is a kind of moxibustion by separating the skin and the moxa cone with drugs. The commonly adopted drugs include the Chinese garlic, ginger and aconite root. Moxibustion with ginger is conducted by applying a ginger slice of 2-3 mm in thickness between the skin and the moxa cone and then lighting the cone. The cone should be fully burnt before it is changed, and the treatment should be continued until the the cones that should be applied are finished. This moxibustion is considered proper when the skin becomes red but no blister occurs. It is usually used to treat vomiting, abdominal pain and diarrhea caused by exposure to cold. The moxibustion with Chinese garlic, conducted in the same way as mentioned above, are mainly used to treat tuberculosis of the lymph glands, lung tuberculosis, etc. The moxibustion with a piece of aconite root (the piece is prepared by grinding the aconite root into powder, mixing the powder with alcohol and then making the mixure to be a piece 30 mm in diameter and 8 mm in thickness) should be conducted in the same way as the moxibustion with ginger, and is mostly used to treat impotence or premature ejaculation.

2. Moxibustion with moxa roll

Moxa roll is made by spreading 24g of mugwort floss over a rough straw paper that is 26 cm in length and 20 cm in width and then rolling up the paper into a cylinde 1. 5 cm in diameter. If the mugwort floss is mixed with such drugs as cassia bark or cloves, it is also called drug roll. Moxibustion with moxa roll can be divided into two kinds: Warming moxibustion and bird-pecking moxibustion.

(1) Warming moxibustion: This is one kind of moxibustion to scorch the acupoint or the diseased area with the ignited end of the moxa roll at a distance of 2-3 cm from the skin to produce a sensation of warmth in the affected part or the acupoint. It is considered proper when patient feels hot with redness of the skin but no burning pain occurs. This treatment should last 5-7 minutes at one point and is mainly applied to treatment of chronic diseases.

(2) Bird-pecking moxibustion: This is one kind of moxibustion conducted by moving the ignited moxa roll up and down instead of fixing the roll at a certain distance from the skin, like a bird pecking food. It is mostly applied to acute diseases.

3. Moxibustion for health care

This means to apply moxibustion when one is healthy to keep health and prevent aging or disease by enhancing the resistant ability against diseases. The commonly used acupoints and methods are as follows:

(1) Moxibustion on Qihai (RN 6): Qihai (RN 6) is an important point for keeping health. Repeated application of moxibustion on this point has the function of building up the primordial Qi, benefiting the Kidney and consolidating the essence. The moxibustion methods commonly applied include warming moxibustion with moxa roll, moxibustion with ginger and moxibustion with aconite piece. Moxibustion at this point is contraindicated for pregnant woman.

(2) Moxibustion on Guanyuan (RN 4): Guanyuan (RN 4) is also an important point for keeping health, which functions to build up the primordial Qi, consolidate the life basis, benefit the Kidney, consolidate the essence and regulate the function of the Chong and Ren Channels. The commonly adopted moxibustions on this point include warm moxibustion with a moxa roll, moxibustion with ginger and moxibustion with aconite root. Moxibustion at this point is contraindicated for pregnant woman.

(3) Moxibustion on Zusanli (ST 36): Zusanli (ST 36), an important point for keeping health, has the function of supporting the Vital Qi, building up the primordial Qi, strengthening the Spleen, regulating the function of the Stomach and harmonizing Qi and

Blood. Moxibustion on this point is applicable to prevention of cerebrovascular disease, and it is mostly used in combination with moxibustion on Juegu (GB 39). Usually the moxibustion with scar formation is adopted.

(4) Moxibustion on Fengmen (BL 12): Moxibustion on Fengmen (BL 12) has the effect of facilitating flow of the Lung Qi, relieving exterior syndrome, expelling Wind and activating collaterals, mostly applied to prevention of common cold. Usually the moxibustion with ginger is adopted.

In additon, moxibustion on Shenque (RN 8), Dazhui (DU 14) and Gaohuang (BL 43) and the moxibustion in summer day also serve as the moxibustion for healthy care.

4. Brief introduction to other moxibustions

(1) Needle warming through moxibustion: This is a kind of moxibustion by applying acupuncture and moxibustion jointly, suitable for diseases that need to be needled with the needle retained and moxibusted. It is carried out by kneading the mugwort floss to the end of needle or sheathing the handle of the needle with a segment of the moxa roll (2 cun or so) after the feeling of gaining Qi is obtained following insertion of needle and proper reinforcing or reducing manipulations are done, then ingiting the roll and when the the moxa floss or the moxa roll is fully burnt, removing the ashes and withdrawing the needle.

(2) Moxibustion with rush pith: This is performed by igniting a rush pith soaked in seasame oil and then applying it to the acupoint that is to be treated to allow the rush pith to explode there. It has the function of dispelling Wind, relieving exterior syndrome, promoting flow of Qi, dissolving Phlegm, freshing the mind and arresting convulsion, mostly used to treat infantile convulsion, coma, stomachache, abdominal pain, etc.

Scalp Acupuncture, Auricular Acupuncture and Electro-acupuncture

1. Scalp acupuncture

Scalp acupunture is a therapy for prevention and treatment of disease by applying acupuncture on specific regions of the scalp. It is mostly adopted to treat cerebral diseases.

(1) Location, action and indication of the commonly used scalp acupuncture lines (MS):

① Middle line of the vertex (MS 5): This refers to the midline of the head from Baihui (DU 20) to Qianding (DU 21), which functions to dredge channels and collaterals, lift Yang, supplement Qi, suppress the Liver and relieve endogenous Wind. It is indicated for diseases of the loins, legs and feet such as paralysis, numbernss, pain, cortical polyuria, prolapse of retum, hypertension, pain in the vertex and infantile enuresis.

② Anterior oblique line of vertex-temporal (MS 6): This is an oblique line drawing from Qianshencong, 1 cun anterior to Baihui (DU 20), which functions to dredge channels and collaterals. It is indicated for contralateral paralysis of the body, contralateral central facial paralysis, aphemia, salivation, and dysphonia.

③ Posterior oblique line of vertex-temporal (MS 7): This is the oblique line drawing from Baihui (DU 20) to Qubin (GB 7), which functions to dredge channels and collaterals. It is indicated for abnormal sensation in the head or the body.

④ Lateral line 1 of vertex (MS 8): This line is 1.5 cun lateral to the midline of the vertex, 1.5 cun from Chengguang (BL 6) backward along the Gallbladder Channel. It functions to dredge channels and collaterals and is indicated for diseases of the loins, legs and feet, such as paralysis, numbness and pain in the lower limbs.

⑤ Lateral line 2 of vertex (MS 9): This line is 2.25 cun lateral to midline of vertex, 1.5 cun from Zhengying (GB 17) backward along the Gallbladder Channel. It functions to dredge channels and collaterals, and is indicated for diseases of the shoulder, the arm and the hand such as paralysis, numbness and pain of the upper limbs.

⑥ Anterior temporal line (MS 10): This is the line connecting Hanyan (GB 4) and Xuanli (GB 6), which functions to dredge channels and collaterals. It is indicated for migrain, aphemia, peripheral facial paralysis and mouth diseases.

⑦ Posterior temporal line (MS 11): This is the line connecting Shuaigu (GB 8) and Qubin (GB 7), which functions to dredge channels and collaterals, improve hearing and relieve vertigo. It is indicated for migrain, dizziness, vertigo and deafness.

⑧ Upper-middle line of occiput (MS 12): This is the line drawing from Qiangjian (DU 18) to Naohu (DU 17), which functions to improve eyesight and strengthen the loins. It is indicated for eye diseases and pain in the lower back.

⑨ Lower-lateral line of occiput (MS 14): This is a vertical line drawing from Yuzhen (BL 9) to the point 2 cun below, which functions to dredge channels and collaterals and calm the Wind. It is indicated for dysequilibrium caused by diseases of the cerebellum, pain in the occipital region, etc.

⑩ Lateral line 1 of forehead (MS 2): This is a line 1 cun from Meichong (BL 3) straight down along the Bladder Channel, which functions to facilitate flow of the Lung Qi, relieve asthma, dissolve Phlegm, arrest cough and tranquilize the mind. It is indicated for diseases of the Upper-Jiao such as diseases of the lung, diseases of the trachea and diseases of the heart.

⑪ Lateral line 2 of forehead (MS 3): This is a line 1 cun from Toulinqi (GB 15) straight down along the Bladder Channel, which functions to strengthen the Spleen, regulate function of the Stomach, relieve stagnation of the Liver Qi and promote flow of Qi. It is indicated for diseases of the Middle-Jiao such as diseases of the spleen, the stomach, the liver, the gallbladder and the pancreas.

⑫ Lateral line 3 of forehead (MS 4): This is a 1 cun long line that is 0.75 cun medial to Touwei (ST 8) straight down along the Stomach Channel, which functions to tonify the Kidney, supplement essence, clear away Heat and remove Dampness. It is indicated for diseases of the Lower-Jiao such as diseases of Kidney or the Bladder and diseases of the urinary or the reproductive systems.

(2) Manipulating method: Ask patient to take a sitting or a lying position. Select the lines in accordance with different diseases. After sterilizing the local areas with routine method, insert a 1. 5-2 cun long filiform needle quickly into the subscapular region at the angle of 30°. When the tip of the needle reaches lower layer of the galea aponeurotica, a decrease of resistance will be felt. Then insert the needle further while twisting and rotating the needle 0. 5-1. 4 cun with the needle being parallel to the scalp. After that, rotate and twist the needle constantly at a frequency of 200 times per minute for 2-3 minutes. Then, retain the needle for 5-10 minutes, during which the needle is manipulated 2-3 times, then withdraw the needle. The manual manipulation may also be replaced by the electro-needling stimuli. In most cases, the treatment should be performed once every day or once every other day, and ten treatments form one course of treatment. The second course is usually resumed 5-7 days later after the first treatment.

(3) Attentions: The stimulation strength must be well mastered in order to prevent faint during acupuncture treatment.

Press the hole of needling for a while following withdrawal of the needle to prevent bleeding.

Patients with acute cerebral bleeding shouldn't be treated with this method until their conditions and their blood pressures stablize. The patients complicated by high fever and cardiac failure shouldn't be treated with this therapy.

2. Auricular acupuncture therapy

This is a method of preventing and treating disease by stimulating the acupoints of the auricle with needling or other methods. It has a wide indication and is easy to perform. Besides, it can be used as an anelgetic method in surgical operation or as a reference for diagnosis of diseases.

(1) Distributing law of the auricular points: The distribution of the auricaulr points have some laws to follow. Generally speaking,

the auricaulr points corresponding to the head or the face are mainly distributed in the lobule; these corresponding to the upper limbs are mainly distributed in the scapha; these corresponding to the trunk and the lower limbs are mainly distributed in the body of the natihelix crus and the superior and the inferior antihelix cruses; these corresponding to the internal organs are mainly distributed in the cymba conchae and the cavum conchae; and these corresponding to the digestive tract are distributed cyclically around the helix crus.

(2) Locations and indications of the commonly used auricular points:

① Upper Jaw (EP-A7): At the midpoint of the region 3 of the lobe; indicated for pain of the upper teeth and tempomanidibular pain.

② Lower Jaw (EP-A5): At the midpoint of the transverse line in the upper part of the region 3 of the lobe; indicated for pain in the lower teeth and pain in the lower jaw joint.

③ Eye (EP-A10): At the center of the region 5 of the lobe; indicated for acute conjunctivitis, electric ophthalmia, and myopia.

④ Internal ear (EP-A12): Slightly above the center of the region 6 of the lobe; indicated for tinnitus, decline of hearing, otitis media, insomnia and auriditary vertigo.

⑤ Adrenal Gland (EP-B8): At the tip of the prominence, inferior to tragus; indicated for hypotension, faint, pulseless syndrome, cough, asthma, common cold, sun-stroke, malaria and mastitis.

⑥ Phargnx and largnx (EP-B4): At the upper 1/2 portion of the inner surface of tragus; indicated for pharyngitis, laryngitis and tonislitis.

⑦ Internal Nose (EP-B6): At the lower 1/2 of the inner durface of the tragus, below the pharynx and the larynx; indicated for rhinitis, accessory nasal sinusitis and common cold.

⑧ Endocrine (EP-D1): At the fundus of interior of concha, interior to intertragic notch; indicated for dysfunction of the urinary or reproductive systems such as menopausal syndrome and skin disorders.

⑨ Occiput (EP-E5): At the posterior and superior corner of the

110

lateral aspect of antitragus; indicated for diseases of the nervous system, skin diseases, coma, occipital pain and insomnia.

⑩Pingchuan (EP-E7): At the tip of the antitragus; indicated for chronic bronchitis, bronchial asthma, mumps, enuresis and acute infantile convulsion.

⑪Forehead (EP-E9): At the anterior-inferior corner of the lateral aspect of antitragus; indicated for pain in the forehead, dizziness, insomnia and heaviness of head.

⑫Subcortex (EP-E10): In the interior aspect of the antitragus; indicated for insomnia, dream-disturbed sleep, pains, poor development of intelligence, asthma, dizziness and tinnitus.

⑬Taiyang (EP-E11): On the lateral aspect of the tragus, between the Occiput and the Forehead; indicated for migrain.

⑭Neck (EP-F5): At the tragic notch, distal to the scapha; indicated for stiff neck, sprain of the cervical muscles, and simple goiter.

⑮Chest (EP-F6): At the antihelix, level with the supratragic notch; indicated for pain in the chest and hypochondrium and mastitis.

⑯Abdomen (EP-F7): At the antihelix, at the level of the lower border of the inferior antihelix crus; indicated for diseases of the abdominal cavity, diseases of the digestive tract and women's diseases.

⑰Toe (EP-G1): At the lateral superior corner of the superior antihelix crus; indicated for numbness and pain of the toes.

⑱Ankle (EP-G3): At the medial superior antihelix crus; indicated for arthritis and sprain and contusion of the ankle joint.

⑲Knee (EP-G4): At the emerging part of the superior antihelix crus, at the level with the upper border of the inferior antihelix crus; indicated for arthritis of the knee joint.

⑳Sympathesis (EP-H1): At the antihelix, on the junction between the termination of the inferior antihelix crus and the helix; indicated for dysfunction of the digestive and the circulatory systems, acute convulsion and dysmenorrhea.

㉑Sciatic Nerve (EP-H2): At the inner 1/2 of the inferior antihelix crus; indicated for sciatica.

111

㉒Shenmen (EP-I1): At the lateral 1/3 of the triangular fossa and anterior to the bifurcation of the inferior and superior antihelix cruses; indicated for insomnia, restlessness, inflammation, asthma, cough, dizziness and urticaria.

㉓Uterus (EP-I 5): At the midpoint of the medial border of helix in the triangular fossa; indicated for irregular menstruation, excessive leukorrhea, dysmenorrhea, pelvic inflammation, impotence and nocturnal emission.

㉔Finger (EP-J1): Above the helix tubercle and the top of the scapha; indicated for numbness and pain of fingers.

㉕Shoulder (EP-J4) At the scapha, level with the supratragic notch; indicated for periarthritis of the shoulder and stiff neck.

㉖Elbow (EP-J5): Between the Wrist and the Shoulder; indicated for pain of the elbow.

㉗Wrist (EP-J6): At the scapha, level with the prominence of the helix tubercle; indicated for pain of the wrist.

㉘Urticaria Region (EP-J10): Between Finger and Wrist; indicated for urticaria and allergic diseases.

㉙Helix 1-6 (EP-K1-6): These are the points formed by dividing the Helix area from the lower border of the helix tubercle to the lower border of the middle part of the lobe into five equal parts (6 points); indicated for fever, infection of the upper respiratory tract, tonsilitis and hypertension.

㉚Ear Apex (EP-K12): At the upper tip of the ear when the helix is folded toward the tragus; indicated for fever, hypertension and stye.

㉛External Genitalia (EP-K13): At the helix, level with the lower border of the inferior antihelix crus; indicated for impotence, inflammation of the external genitals, and skin disorders of the perineum.

㉜Lower Portion of Retum (EP-K15): At the helix, level with the Large Intestine; indicated for constipation, dysentery, prolapse of rectum and hemorrhoids.

㉝Mouth (EP-M1): In the superior and posterior border of the opening of the external auditary canal; indicated for facial paralysis and stomatitis.

㉞Esophagus (EP-M2): At the inner 2/3 inferior to the helix crus; indicated for nausea, vomiting, and dysphagia.

㉟Cardia (EP-M3): At the posterior 1/3 inferior to the helix crus; indicated for nausea, vomiting and cardiospasm.

㊱Stomach (EP-M4): In the area where the helix crus terminates; indicated for hiccup, vomiting, indigestion, gastric ulcer and insomnia.

㊲Duodenum (EP-M5): At the lateral 1/3 above the helix crus; indicated for diseases of the biliary tract, duodenal ulcer and cardiospasm.

㊳Small Intestine (EP-M6): At the middle 1/3 superior to the helix crus; indicated for indigestion and palpitation.

㊴Large Intestine (EP-M8): At the inner 1/3 above the helix crus; indicated for dysentery, diarrhea and constipation.

㊵Appendix (EP-M7): Between Small Intestine and Large Intestine; indicated for appendicitis and diarrhea.

㊶Kidney (EP-N4): In the lower border of the inferior antihelix crus, directly above Small Intestine; indicated for diseases of the urinary system and reproductive system, the women's diseases, lumbago, tinnitus, insomnia, hypertrophy of the cervical and the lumbar vertebrae.

㊷Pancreas, Gallbladder (EP-N6): Between the Liver and the Kidney in the superior concha of the right and the left ear respectively; indicated for pancratitis, diabetes, diseases of the biliary tract, migraine and malaria.

㊸Liver (EP-N9): At the superior concha, posterior to Stomach and Duodenum; indicated for eye diseases, malaria, irregular menstruation, dysmenorrhea and hypochondriac pain.

㊹Spleen (EP-N10): Inferior to Liver, at the lateroinferior aspect of the superior concha; indicated for indigestion, chronic diarrhea, stomachache, stomatitis, metrostaxis and metrorrhagia and hemopathy.

㊺Heart (EP-O1): In the center of inferior concha; indicated for diseases of the cardiovascular diseases, sun-stroke and acute convulsion.

㊻Lung (EP-O2): In the superior, inferior and lateral sides of Heart; indicated for diseases of the respiratory system, skin diseases and common cold.

㊼Trachea (EP-O4):Between the Mouth and the Heart; indicated for cough and asthma.

㊽Triple-Jiao (EP-O5): At the inferior concha, superior to Endocrine; indicated for constipation and edema.

㊾Groove of Blood Pressure-Lowering (EP-Z1): In the back of ear, a depression distributed from the medial superior side to the lateral inferior side; indicated for hypertension.

㊿Upper Ear Back (EP-Z2): At the prominence of the cartilage in the upper part of the back of ear; indicated for skin diseases, headache, sciatica and lumbago.

51Lower Ear Back (EP-Z4): At the prominence of the cartilage of the back of ear; indicated for skin diseases, cough, pain in the back and asthma.

52Middle Ear Back (EP-Z3): At the highest point between the Upper Ear Back and the Lower Ear Back; indicated for skin diseases, pain in the back, abdominal fullness, diarrhea and indigestion.

(3) Principles for selection and prescription of the auricular points: This mainly includes: The slection of the auricular points in accordance with syndrome, which means to select the points related to the syndromes identified in the light of the Zang-Fu theory and the meridian theory of TCM, for example, skin diseases may be treated by selecting the point Lung because, in accordance with TCM theory, the Lung is related to the skin; Selection of the auricular points in accordance with symptoms, which means to select the auricular points in the light of the physiology and pathology of Western medicine, for example, menstrual diseases may be treated by selecting the Endocrine; Selection of the auricular points in accordance with diseases, which means to select the auricular points in the light of diagnosis of disease, for example, the Stomach point may be selected for treating stomach diseases; and expirical selec-

114

tion of the auricular points, which means to select the effective auricular points for some diseases in the light of the clinical practice,
for example, the Ear Center point can be chosen to treat hemopathy
and skin disease, and the Stomach point to treat diseases of the nervous system.

(4) Manipulating methods: When the auricular points are selected
in the light of the diseases, they must be strictly sterilized. Then,
select a 0.5 cun long short filiform needle or special thumbtack-
shape needle. When inserting the filiform needle, doctor, with the
left hand fixing the ear, inserts the needle into the cartilage with his
right hand. The tip of the needle shouldn't penetrate the skin on the
opposite side. The thumbtack needles should be fixed to the skin
with plaster when they are inserted into the auricular points. There
are also such sensations as hotness, numbness or transmission along
the channels. The filiform needle is usually retained for 10-20 minutes, but for cases with painful symptoms, it may be retained for 1-
2 hours or more, during which the needle may be manipulated intermittently. The thumbtack needle may be retained for 2-3 days in the
spring and autumn, and 7-10 days in winter. But it shouldn't be retained too long in summer. During the retaining of the needle, patient should press the needles, 1-3 minutes each time, 2-3 times a
day. When the needle is withdrawn, the hole should be pressed a
while with a dry sterilized cotton ball to prevent bleeding. If necessary, the holes should be sterilized with commonly used method a-
gain to prevent infection. Usually, the acute diseases should be
treated 1-2 times a day, and the chronic diseases, once a day or once
every other day, with 10 days as a course of treatment. The second
course of treatment usually begins at an interval of 5-7 days.

(5) Attentions: The skin to be punctured must be strictly sterilized in order to prevent infection, and the skin with infection or the
frozen area are contraindicated for needling. If there is redness of
the hole of needling and distending pain of the ear, which indicate
mild infection, iodine alcohol should be applied to the affected area
immediately, three times a day, and the Liver point or the Shenmen
point should be punctured, or the antibiotics should be given. Be

115

sure not to cause pyogenic perichondritis of the ear.

Faint must be noted carefully since auricular acpuncture give rises to severe pain.

The senile patients and the patients with general weakness should rest some time before and after the needling. Pregnant woman with a history of habitual abortion is contraindicated for ear needling.

If the pyogenic perichondritis of the ear occurs, it may be treated by performing warming moxibustion with an ignited moxa roll, 15-30 minutes each time, three times daily, until the disease is cured. If there is pus formation, the pus must be drainaged thoroughly by exlarging the wound before moxibustion is applied, and antibiotics should be given at the same time.

3. The electric acupuncture therapy

This is a method to prevent and treat disease by connecting the needle with the electron in a small volume of electrical current accessory to that of the human body following the feeling of gaining Qi is obtained. As its merits, this therapy can enhance the therapeutic effects on some diseases by combining the effect of the needling and the effect of the impulse electric current, the stimulation parameters are easy to master, and it can take the place of the manual manipulation of the needles.

(1) Slection of the electric acunpuncture instruments: The instruments for electric acupunctures are various. The popularly adopted at present is that made up of the transister parts which perform its effect by means of the low frequencies current accessory to bio-electricity of the human body produced by an oscillation producer. The electric acupuncture instrument should be able to produce a strong stimuli, safety, not limited by the electric source, small in volume, easy to carry out and resistant to vibration. It should also work under the support of dry battery, consume less electricity and produce no noise.

(2) Operating method: The output potentiometer must be adjusted to be "Zero" before the use of the electric acupuncture instrument. Then, connects each pair of the output voltage wire with the handles of two filiform needles and then turn the switch to select the

116

required waves and frequencies. After that, increase gradually the output electric current to what is needed to produce a sourness and distending sensation or rhythmic contraction of the muscles that patient can tolerate. The stimuli should increase properly, or the waves or frequency should be changed in patient who may get adaptive to the stimuli in the case of being treated with this method for a long time, in order to maintain the necessary effect. After treatment, adjust the output potentiometer to be "Zero" first, then turn the switch to "off", take away the wire from the needles, and withdraw the needles. One electric acupuncture treatment usually lasts 5-20 minutes, but it may last a longer time if it is used for anaesthesia or pains.

(3) Indications: The electric acupuncture therapy has wide indications, which are basically the same with those of the acupuncture with filiform needles. Clinically, it is applied to pains, paralysis, dysfunction of the heart, the stomach, the intestine, the gallbladder, the bladder and the uterus, epilepsy, schizophrenia, and injury to the muscles, ligaments or joints. It can also be used for acupuncture anaesthesia.

As the waves applied are different, the therapeutic effects are also different. It is usually believed that the intensive wave can lower the stress function of the nervous syetm, causing inhibiting response, mostly used to relieve pain, sedate the mind, alleviate the spasm of muscles and vessels or for acupuncture anaesthesia. The sparse wave can enhance the tension of the muscles and ligaments, so it has an obvious exciting effect and thus is mainly adopted to treat paralysis and injury to the muscles, joints, ligaments and tendons; the sparse-intensive waves can promote circulation and metabolism of blood, improve the nutrition of tissues and remove inflammatory edema, therefore, it is mainly used to arrest pain and relieve inflammation; and the intermittent waves have a better stimulating effect on promoting contraction, so it is often adopted to treat paralysis or myoasthenia.

(4) Attentions: Before treatment, careful examination on the electric acupuncture instrument must be done to see whether it

works well or not.

The output voltage of the electric acupuncture instrument must be kept less than 40 V and the output current should be less than 1 mA, in order to prevent patient from getting an electric shock.

The electric current should be adjusted gradully from small to large. Sudden increase must be avoided lest it cause violent contraction of muscles and the ensuing faint during acupuncture, bending or breaking of the needles.

The current loop should not pass through the heart in patients with cardiac diseases. When the instrument is applied to the medulla or spine, the current must be small, and pregnant woman should be treated with this instrument very carefully.

A General Introduction to the Acupuncture- Moxibustion Therapeutics

A cupuncture-moxibustion therapeutics is a speciality dealing with how to apply such basic theories, basic knowledge and basic skills as the basic theory of TCM, the meridian theory, the acupoint theory and the acupuncture-moxibustion therapy in the clinical practice to prevent and treat diseases. It is an important component of the acupuncture-moxibustion science.

The acupuncture-moxibustion treatment is a process in which the causes and pathogenesis of a disease, the locations of disease (Zang organs, Fu organs, exterior or interior), the natures of disease (Cold, Heat, Excess or Deficiency) and the urgency of the fundamental cause of disease and the manifestations of disease, are firstly identified by summarizing and analysing the data gained throught the four diagnostic techniques of TCM in accordance with the Zang-Fu theory, the meridian theory, and the eight principles for syndrome identification. Then, in the light of the results of syndrome identification, formulate the prescriptions of acupoints and apply the acupuncture therapy, the moxibustion therapy or the combined

119

acupuncture-moxibustion therapy with reducing method, reinforcing method or the uniform reinforcing and reducing method, with an aim to drege the channels and collaterals, regulate Qi and Blood, restore balance between Yin and Yang and harmonize the function of Zang-Fu organs by which to prevent and treat disease and keep one's health.

Statistics shows that acupuncture-moxibustion is effective for more than 300 kinds of diseases, and better or highly effective therapeutic effects can be achieved in about 100 kinds of diseases. In China, acupuncture anaesthesia has been adopted in the surgical operation of more than 100 kinds of diseases.

Mechanism of Acupuncture-Moxibustion Therapy

1. Regulating Yin and Yang

TCM believes that the primary causes of all diseases are that Yin and Yang of the human body lose their equilibrium and Excess or Deficiency of Yin or Yang occurs as a result. Acupuncture-moxibustion cures disease by using points in joint and the different manipulations of needles to adjust the Excess or Deficiency of Yin or Yang and restore the physiological balance between Yin and Yang.

2. Supporting Vital Qi and eliminating pathogens

From the viewpoint of the pathogen and Vital Qi, the process of occurrence and development of disease is in fact a process in which pathogen and Vital Qi fight against each other. The Vital Qi refers to various kinds of substances maintaing the life energy and functions as well as the resistant ability of the human body against disease produced by these substances or functions. The so-called pathogen is a general term for all the pathogenic factors. Result of the struggle between the Vital Qi and the pathogen determines the prognosis of a disease. Practice proves that acupuncture with reinforcing manipulations on the selected points has the function of supporting the Vital Qi, while that with reducing manipulations on selected points has the effect of eliminating pathogens. So, acupuncture-moxibustion works through supporting the Vital Qi and eliminating the pathogens so that the Vital Qi will win in the struggle and disease will turn to be mild or cured.

3. Dredging the channels and collaterals

Channels and collaterals are the passageways which connect the five Zang organs and the six Fu organs with the superficial tissues and organs such as the muscles, the skins, the sensory organs, the nine orifices and the limbs. They have the functions of communicating with and connecting with the Zang-Fu organs and the limbs, circulating Qi and Blood and nourishing the whole body. Once Qi and Blood in the channels and collaterals lose their harmony, they will become excessive or deficient in the channels and collaterals, leading to adverse flow and stagnation of Qi and Blood, and the ensuing occurrence of various kinds of diseases. In such a case, application of different acupuncture-moxibustion therapy at acupoints or channels can play a therapeutic role by regulating Qi and Blood, removing the stagnancy, reinforcing the Deficiency and purging the Excess.

4. Regulating the functional states of Zang-Fu organs

Man is an organic unity in which the different Zang-Fu organs coordinate with and assist each other in physiology. When disease occurs in a Zang or a Fu organ, it often involves the functional activities of other Zang-Fu organs through the channels and collaterals. Acupuncture-moxibustion, through regulating the relationships of Zang-Fu organs, can harmonize the functions of the Zang-Fu organs and thus treat disease with better therapeutic effects.

Therapeutic Principles of Acupuncture-Moxibustion

The therapeutic principles adopted in acupuncture-moxibustion therapy are dependent upon the natures of diseases, which can be generalized as Yin or Yang, exterior or interior, Cold or Heat, and Deficiency or Excess, though they may be very complicated.

1. Yin and Yang

Generally speaking, diseases of the exterior of the body or Fu organs with a Heat or an Excess nature belong to Yang; while these of the interior of the body or the Zang organ with a Cold or a Deficiency nature belong to Yin. Clinically, diseases of a Yang nature are mainly manifested as excessive Heat syndrome, so they should be treated with reducing method or a rapid inserting method or with pricking method to cause bleeding; while these of a Yin nature, are mostly manifested as Deficiency Cold syndrome and thus should be treated with reducing method with the needle retained, or by moxibustion therapy. This is the basic principle for acupuncture-moxibustion treatment of diseases.

2. Exterior and interior

Exterior and interior usually indicate the depth of diseases. Diseases located in the channels and collaterals, skin or muslces belong to the exterior and should be treated by needling superficially with quick withdrawal of the needle; while these in the Zang or Fu organs, tendons and bones belong to interior and should be treated by deep needling and long retaining of needle. As for the exterior syndrome caused by exogenous pathogens, reducing method should be applied in acupuncture, moxibustion or combined use of acupuncture and moxibustion treatments. If the pathogen enters the interior and affects Zang-Fu organs, acupuncture or moxibustion therapy with reinforcing or reducing method or combined use of acupuncture and moxibustion therapies should be adopted, depending on the different situations.

3. Cold and Heat

In most cases, Cold syndromes arise from Excess of Yin Qi or Deficiency of Yang Qi of the human body. So, different methods such as acupuncture therapy, moxibustion therapy and combined acupuncture and moxibustion therapies, should be adopted with different manipulations such as the reinforcing manipulation, the reducing manipulation and the uniform reinforcing and reducing manipulations, in accordance with the position of the Cold pathogen (on the exterior or the interior) and the nature of the disease (Deficiency or Excess). Yang syndrome are mostly caused by Excess of Yang Qi or Deficiency of the Yin-Fluid of the human body, and are usually treated by rapid needling with reducing method or by pricking to cause bleeding. Moxibustion cannot be applied.

4. Deficiency and Excess

Deficiency and Excess indicate vicissitude of the Vital Qi and the waning and waxing of pathogens. Deficiency syndromes include all the diseases caused by Deficiency of the Vital Qi, including Deficiency of Yin, Deficiency of Yang, Deficiency of Zang-Fu organs, Deficiency of meridians and Deficiency of Qi and Blood, so they should be treated with reinforcing method in the acupuncture treatment or by both acupuncture and moxibustion treatments. Excess syndromes indicate exuberance of pathogens or hyperactivities of the human body, so they should be treated with reducing method or by pricking to cause bleeding, in order to eliminate the excessive pathogens. As for diseases of Deficiency complicated by Excess or these of Excess complicated by Deficiency, they may be treated by the reinforcing method first followed by reducing method or vice versa, or both the reducing and reinforcing methods in accordance with difference of the severity of the Excess and Deficiency.

Principles for Slection of Points and Prescriptions in Acupuncture-Moxibustion Treatment

As acupuncture-moxibustion treats disease by needling or moxi-busting some acupoints of the human body, selection of the acupoints, and the prescriptions have a close relationship with the therapeutic effects.

1. Basic laws of acupuncture-moxibustion prescriptions formulation

The selection of acupoints in acupuncture-moxibustion treatment is conducted under the guidance of the meridian theory in accordance with different diseases, with selection of acupoint along the distribution of channels as the main law.

(1) Selection of the local points: This is based on the law that each of the acupoints can treat diseases of the area where the acupoint is located and these of the area adjacent to the acupoint, used mostly to treat superficial diseases with markable symptoms or localized superficial diseases. It is a widely applied method. For example, diseases of the nose can be treated by selecting Yingxiang (LI 20).

(2) Selection of the remote points: This is a method to select the points suggested based on such basic theories of TCM as the theory of Yin and Yang, the theory of Zang-Fu organs and the theory of meridians. Clinically, a disease can be treated by selecting both the points on the channel pertaining to the diseased Zang-Fu organ and the points of the interior-exteriorly related channel or other related channels. For example, stomachache can be treated with Zusanli (ST 36), Gongsun (SP 3), Taichong (LR 3) and Neiguan (PC 6), which is just a concrete application of this method.

(3) Selection of points in accordance with syndromes: Different from the selection of the local points and the selection of the remote

124

points, this method is suggested based on the basic theory of TCM and the actions and indications of acupoints. It is mainly applicable to general diseases of the human body such as fever, spontaneous sweating, night sweating, insomnia and collapse. If the selection of the local points and the selection of the remote points cannot cover the treatment of all the manifestations of disease, this method should be adopted. For example, fever in exogenous diseases can be treated by selecting Dazhui (DU 14), Hegu (LI 4) and Quchi (LI 11).

The above three methods may be adopted alone or jointly in the clinic, which also serves as a basic law that must be followed in formulating a prescription of acupuncture-moxibustion.

2. The law of changes of prescriptions

Although the same point may be included in different prescriptions, it may bring about different therapeutic effects in different situations as a result of the difference in its manipulations (reinforcing or reducing), order of needling, the acupoints used in combination, the depth of needling for the point and whether the needle is retained at the point or not. This is also a basic law of changes of the acupoint prescriptions concerning their therapeutic effects, which is discussed in detail as follows.

(1) Difference of the reinforcing and the reducing effects: Reinforcing and reducing methods in acupuncture-moxibustion treatments are completely opposite in their manipulations and therapeutic effects. As a result, the same point in different prescriptions may give rise to completely different effects. For example, reinforcing Hegu (LI 4) and reducing Sanyinjiao (SP 6) can promote flow of Qi, remove Blood Stasis, activate channels and dissipate Blood Stasis, but if Hegu (LI 4) is needled with a reducing method and Sanyinjiao (SP 6) with a reinforcing method, it will have the function of regulating flow of Qi, enriching Blood and consolidating Blood in the channels to treat dysfunctional uterine bleeding.

(2) Difference of the depth of the needling: Depth of needling also has a close relationship with the therapeutic effects of the prescription. In the clinic, as the depth of needling is different, the thera-

peutic effects of an acupoint may be obviously different. Therefore, one must take the different effects produced by needling different depths into consideration, so that he can apply the different methods flexibly in the light of the different diseases, different times and different patients.

(3) Different roles of acupoints in prescription and the different order of needling: Acupoints in one prescription may play a leading role or a supplementary role, and they may be inserted first or later. The difference in inserting the needles into different points may give rise to different therapeutic effects. Usually the acupoints in the upper part or of the Yang channels are needled first, then these in the lower part or of the Yin channels. In some special conditions, the order may be adjusted in accordance with the patients' conditions, in order to achieve a better therapeutic effects.

(4) Different roles of acupuncture-moxibustion in treating different diseases: The acupuncture and moxibustion have something different from each other, so they should be applied differently in clinic. For example, excessive Heat syndrome is usually treated by acupuncture instead of the moxibustion; while a Deficiency-Cold syndrome is mainly treated with moxibustion instead of acupuncture. So, one must analyze which one of the acupuncture therapy, the moxibustion therapy or the combined acupuncture and moxibustion therapy is more proper for a disease according to the patients' conditions.

(5) Modifications of acupoints in prescription: Increase or reduce of the acupoints in a prescription concerns not only with the therapeutic effects, but also with the indications of the prescription. Generally, a prescription should be modified in accordance with the changes of diseases with the main points remained the same. For example, when Hegu (LI 4) is used together with Quchi (LI 11) with Hegu (LI 4) as the main point, it forms an important prescription for treating diseases in the Upper-Jiao; When Hegu (LI 4) is used together with Sanyinjiao (SP 6) with Hegu as the main point, it forms a prescription with the function of promoting flow of Qi, activating Blood and regulating menstruation; and when Hegu (LI 4) is

126

used together with Fuliu (KI 7) with the Hegu (LI 4) as the main point, it can induce perspiration or arrest sweating. These differences in the therapeutic effects lie in the differences of the modifications of the acupoints.

Commonly Used Methods to Use Acupoints Jointly

Using points jointly means to use the points with the same or similar therapeutic effects simultaneously to achieve a coordinative effect of the actions of the points, which is discussed as follows.

1. Using the points of the same channel

This means that the acupoints of the same channel can be adopted in one prescription to treat the disease of this channel or the disease of the Zang or Fu organ that the channel pertains to.

2. Using the points of the interior-exteriorly related channels jointly

This means to select the acupoints of the diseased channel and these of its interior-exteriorly related channels simultaneously in one prescription to treat diseases of this channel or the diseases of the Zang or Fu organ this channel pertains to.

3. Using the points on the back and the front jointly

The front of the body, referring to the chest and abdomen, is a Yin place; while the back of the body, including the back and the lower back, is a Yang place, so this is a method to form a prescription with both the acupoints on the back and these on the chest and abdomen. Combined use of the Back-Shu point and the Front-Mu point is just such an example.

4. Using the points on the upper part of the body and these on the lower part of the body jointly

The upper part of the body refers to the part above the waist of the body, while the lower part, the part below the waist of the body. So, this is a method to form a prescription with both the acu-points in the upper part of the body and these in the lower part of the body. Combined use of the eight crossing points of the eight ex-traordinary channels is just such an example.

5. Using the points on the left and these on the right jointly

This is a method to form a prescription based on the different portions affected by exogenous pathogens and crossing of channels in their distribution. It may adopt the same point of the bilateral sides to form the prescription, or adopt the points on the left side to treat diseases of the right side or vice versa.

Treatment of Common Diseases with Acupuncture-Moxibustion

Infectious Diseases

1. Influenza

*I*nfluenza is an acute infectious disease of the respiratory tract caused by influenza virus. It is clinically manifested as sudden onset and such actue poisonous symptoms as aversion to cold, fever, headache, general weakness, aching of muscles which is more severe in the muscles of the back and lower back and the gastrocnemius muscle, as well as the symptoms of the respiratory tract. It is highly infectious, tends to spread rapidly, and often becomes epidemic or world-wide pandemic. Mostly, the disease is seen in the spring and winter, but it may also be seen in other seasons. In TCM, it is called epidemic common cold.

(1) Syndrome identification:

① Wind-Cold type: Mild fever with severe chills, headache,

aching of the limbs, stuffy nose, nasal discharge, itching of throat, cough with clear and thin sputum, no sweat, pale tongue with thin and whitish coating and floating rapid pulse.

② Wind-Heat type: Severe fever with mild chills, distending pain of the head, dry nose, sore throat, cough with thick sputum, thirst with a desire for drink, red tongue with thin and yellow coating and floating rapid pulse. If Summer-Heat and Dampness are complicated, there is high fever, sweating which cannot reduce the fever, heaviness of the body, lassitude, yellow and greasy tongue coating and soft rapid pulse. If pathogenic Dryness is complicated, there is fever with mild aversion to cold, dry mouth and throat, red tongue with little coating and a fine and rapid pulse.

(2) Therapeutic methods:

① Wind-Cold type:

Prescription: Lieque (LU 7), Fengmen (BL 12), Fengchi (GB 20) and Hegu (LI 4).

Manipulation: Puncture the above points superficially with filiform needles and with reducing method. Uniform reinforcing and reducing method is adopted in patients with weak constitutions. And, moxibustion may be applied simultaneously.

② Wind-Heat type:

Prescription: Dazhui (DU 14), Quchi (LI 11), Hegu (LI 4), Yuji (LU 10) and Waiguan (SJ 5).

Manipulation: With reducing method, puncture the above points with filiform needles superficially. Add Quze (PC 3), Weizhong (BL 40), Yinlingquan (SP 9) and Zusanli (ST 36) for cases complicated by Summer-Heat and Dampness; and add Taixi (KI 3) and Zhaohai (KI 6) to be needled with reinforcing method for cases complicated by pathogenic Dryness.

(3) Other therapy:

Auricular acupuncture: Lung (EP-O2), Trachea (EP-O4), Forehead (EP-E9), Larynx and Pharynx (EP-B4), Internal Nose (EP-B6), Tonsil (EP-K7-K9). 2-3 points are used each time and the above points are adopted alternately with moderate stimuli. Manipulate the needle for 1-2 minutes and retain the needle for 30-60 minutes with intermittent manipulations of the needles.

2. Epidemic mumps

Epidemic mumps is an acute infectious disease of the respiratory tract caused by mumps virus, which is characterized by non-pyogenic swelling, distending and pain of the parotid gland accompanied by fever and mild discomfort of the body. It may be complicated with mumps meningitis, testis, etc. This disease mostly affects the children from 5 to 15 years old and may be epidemic all the year round, although it is mostly seen in the winter and spring. In TCM, it is called Zha Sai (Swollen cheeks).

(1) Syndrome identification:

① Syndrome of Wind-warmth: Chills, fever, headache, aching in the region below the ear, difficulty in opening mouth, followed by swelling and pain of the parotid gland with an indistinct border, normal spirit, thin whitish or yellowish tongue coating, and floating and rapid pulse.

② Syndrome of toxic warmth: Chills, high fever, headache, vexation, thirst, anorexia, swelling and pain of the parotid gland with a burning sensation which is aggravated by pressing, dry stools, scanty dark urine, red tongue with thin greasy and yellow coating and a slippery rapid pulse.

③ Testitis secondary to mumps: Mostly seen in children above 12 years old or the adults, marked by sudden high fever, tremor, swelling, distension, pain or a lowering-down sensation of testis or even edema of the scrotum that occur one week after swelling of the parotic gland occurs.

④ Convulsion secondary to mumps: Seen mostly in children, which usually occurs within one week following swelling of the parotic gland, marked by high fever, vomiting, lethargy, signs of meningeal irritation and convulsion.

(2) Therapeutic methods:

① Syndrome of Wind-warmth:

Prescription: Fengchi (GB 20), Yemen (SJ 2), Hegu (LI 4), Waiguan (SJ 5), Yifeng (SJ 17) and Jiache (ST 6).

Manipulations: Reducing with filiform needle.

131

② Syndrome of toxic warmth:

Prescription: Add Quchi (LI 11) and Fenglong (ST 40) to the above prescription.

Manipulation: Puncture with filiform needle, reducing method and strong stimuli.

③ Testitis secondary to mumps:

Prescription: Add Taichong (LR 3), Sanyinjiao (SP 6) and Xuehai (SP 10) to the prescription for syndrome of Wind-warmth.

Manipulation: Puncture with filiform needles and reducing method.

④ Convulsion secondary to mumps:

Prescription: Shixuan (EX-UE 11), Hegu (LI 4), Taichong (LR 3), Yanglingquan (GB 34), Shuigou (DU 26) and Dazhui (DU 14).

Manipulation: Puncture superfically with filiform needles and reducing method and withdraw the needles quickly without retaining of the needle. Or, prick with a three edged needle to cause bleeding.

(3) Other therapy:

Moxibustion with rush pith: Ignite the rush pith dipped in plant oil and then touch Jiaosun (SJ 20) of the affected side quickly and lightly with the pith to produce a clear and melodious sound like that of a firecracker. The treatment is administered twice a day.

3. Bacterial dysentery

Bacterial dysentery is an infectious diseases of the intestinal tract caused by dysentery bacillus, which mostly occurs in the summer and autumn. The main pathological changes are the diffusive inflammation of the mucosa of the intestine, and clinically, it is marked by fever, abdominal pain, diarrhea, tenesmus and discharge of stools with pus and blood. In TCM, it is named "intestinal hemorrhage", "dysentery" or "pestilent dysentery".

(1) Syndrome identification:

① Syndrome of Dampness-Heat: Abdominal pain, tenesmus, diarrhea with the stool containing pus and blood, burning sensation in the anus, scanty and dark urine, red tongue with yellow and sticky tongue coating and slippery rapid pulse.

② Pestilent dysentery: Sudden onset, high fever, thirst, headache with restlessness, coma in severe cases, or severe abdominal pain, diarrhea with the stool containing bright red or purplish blood and pus, red or crimson tongue with yellow and dry coating and rapid slippery pulse.

③ Dysentery of Cold-Dampness: Diarrhea with stools containing more pus than blood, tenesmus, heaviness of the head and body, pale tongue with sticky coating and soft and moderate pulse.

④ Dysentery with trismus: Fulminant diarrhea, abdominal pain, vomiting right after eating, or stomachache after eating, vomiting, or dry mouth and tongue, nausea, belch, thick and sticky or yellow greasy tongue coating, fine and rapid or slippery rapid pulse.

⑤ Dysentery of Deficiency-Cold: Diarrhea with watery stools containing the pus, abdominal dull pain, poor appetite, listlessness, no thirst, desiring for warmth and aversing to cold, or diarrhea at dawn, pale tongue with thin and whitish coating and fine and weak pulse.

⑥ Recurrent dysentery: Chronic and recurrent diarrhea with pus and blood, tenesmus, pale tongue and weak or slippery wiry pulse.

(2) Therapeutic method:

Prescription: Tianshu (ST 25), Hegu (LI 4), Shangjuxu (ST 37).

Manipulation: Puncture with filiform needles by reducing method. Add Dazhui (DU 14) and Shixuan (EX-UE11) to be pricked to cause bleeding for cases with pestilent dysentery; add Zhongwan (RN 12) and Neiguan (PC 6) for cases with dysentery and trismus; add Yinlingquan (SP 9) and Qihai (RN 6) for cases with dysentery of Cold-Dampness; add Pishu (BL 20) and Shenshu (BL 23) for cases with dysentery of Deficiency-Cold; and add Pishu (BL 20) and Weishu (BL 21) for cases with recurrent dysentery. The above added points except for Dazhui (DU 14) and Shixuan (EX-UE11) are to be treated with reinforcing method.

Diseases of the Internal Medicine

1. Acute tracheobronchitis

This is an acute inflammation of the mucous membrane of the trachea and the bronchus caused by infection, physical or chemical stimuli or allergic response, which is clinically manifested as cough with sputum. It is usually seen in a cold season and is often induced by sudden changes of weather. In TCM, this disease is called "cough".

(1) Syndrome differention:

① Wind-Heat syndrome: Cough with yellow sputum, fever, headache, thin and yellow tongue coating, and floating and rapid pulse.

② Wind-Cold syndrome: Cough with thin, white sputum, itching of throat, headache, fever, aversion to cold, no sweating, thin and whitish tongue coating and floating tense pulse.

③ Dryness-Heat syndrome: Dry cough without sputum, or with scanty and sticky sputum which is difficult to be expectorated, dry nose and throat, red tongue with little fluid, fine and rapid pulse.

(2) Therapeutic methods:

① Wind-Cold syndrome:

Prescription: Lieque (LU 7), Hegu (LI 4), Feishu (BL 13), Waiguan (SJ 5).

Manipulation: Puncture superficially with filiform needles and reducing method and retain the needle.

② Wind-Heat syndrome:

Prescription: Chize (LU 5), Feishu (BL 13), Quchi (LI 11), Dazhui (DU 14).

Manipulation: Puncture quickly with filiform needle and reducing method.

③ Dryness-Heat syndrome:

Prescription: Fengmen (BL 12), Feishu (BL 13), Taiyuan (LU 9), Fuliu (KI 7).

Manipulation: After gaining of feeling of Qi, the needle should be retained for a short time. Except for Fuliu (KI 7), which is treated with reinforcing method, other points should be treated with reducing method.

(3) Other therapy:

Auricular acupuncture: Puncture Trachea (EP-O4), Bronchus (EP-O3), Shenmen (EP-I1) and Occiput (EX-E5) with strong or moderate stimuli, retain the needles for 30 minutes, once daily.

2. Chronic bronchitis

This refers to the non-specific inflammation of the mucous membrane of the trachea and bronchus or their adjacent tissues, which is clinically marked by cough with sputum or accompanied with dyspnea that takes a chronic course with the above symptoms attacking repeatedly. It is mostly seen in the aged and can be diagnosed only when it lasts more than 3 months a year in 2 successive years. In TCM, it is called "cough" or "asthma".

(1) Syndrome identification:

① Phlegm-Dampness syndrome: Cough with an unclear sound, more severe in the morning, profuse thick sputum, white or grey in colour, white and greasy tongue coating and soft or moderate pulse.

② Liver Fire syndrome: Paroxismal attack of cough with little thick sputum, pain in the hypochondrium while coughing, red face, dry throat, bitter taste in the mouth, red tongue tip, thin white coating with little fluid and wiry and rapid pulse.

③ Kidney Deficiency syndrome: Cough with much white and clear sputum, asthma which is aggravated by exertion, soreness and weakness of the loins and knees, frequent urination, white tongue coating with much fluid, and deep, fine and forcelss pulse.

(2) Therapeutic methods:

① Phlegm-Dampness syndrome:

Prescription: Feishu (BL 13), Pishu (BL 20), Taiyuan (LU 9), Taibai (SP 3), Hegu (LI 4) and Fenglong (ST 40).

Manipulation: Puncture with filiform needles and the uniform reinforcing and reducing method. Use reducing method by lifting and inserting the needles in Hegu (LI 4) and Fenglong (ST 40). Moxibustion is added to the acupoints on the back.

② Liver Fire syndrome:

Prescription: Feishu (BL 13), Ganshu (BL 18), Jingqu (LU 8), Taichong (LR 3).

Manipulation: Ganshu (BL 18) and Taiyuan (LR 3) are treated by reducing method with filiform needles; Feishu (BL 13) and Jingqu (LU 8) are treated with uniform reinforcing and reducing method. Moxibustion is not used.

③ Kidney Deficiency syndrome:

Prescription: Shenshu (BL 23), Taixi (KI 3), Taiyuan (LU 9), Guanyuan (RN 4) and Dingchuan (EX-B 1).

Manipulation: The above points are treated with filiform needles by using reinforcing method, moxibustion can be applied to Shenshu (BL 23), Dingchuan (EX-B1) and Guanyuan (RN 4).

(3) Other therapy:

Moxibustion with ginger: This is applied to Dazhui (DU 14), Dingchuan (EX-B 1), Fengmen (BL 12), Feishu (BL 13), Jueyinshu (BL 14) and Xinshu (BL 15) in the hottest day of summer. 3 moxa rolls should be finished at each point each time, and the treatment should be done 3 times a week, 12 times in all.

3. Bronchial asthma

Bronchial asthma is a disease marked by excessive increase of the reactivity of the trachea and bronchus to the stimuli of antibody or non-antibody. It is clinically characterized by expiratory dyspnea with rale sound in the thorat, which lasts from several minutes to several hours or more, after which it may relieve itself or be relieved after treatment. It mostly affects the children below 12 years old, and in TCM, it is called "asthma".

(1) Syndrome identification:

① The Excess syndrome: That caused by attack of exogenous Wind-Cold is marked by cough with clear sputum, aversion to cold, no sweating, headache, absence of thirst, thin and whitish tongue coating and a floating and tense pulse; that caused by Phlegm-Heat is marked by cough with difficulty in expectorating the yellow, stick sputum, chest fullness or fever, thrist, constipation, yellow greasy tongue coating and a slippery rapid pulse.

② The Deficiency syndrome: Marked by dyspnea, feeble voice, perspiration on activity, pale tongue and a fine rapid or feeble pulse, or by listlessness, shortness of breath, dyspnea on activity, sweating, cold limbs and a deep and fine pulse.

(2) Therapeutic methods:

① The Excess syndrome:

Prescription: Shanzhong (RN 17), Lieque (LU 7), Feishu (BL 13), Chize (LU 5).

Manipulation: The above points are treated with reducing method by filiform needles. For the case due to Wind-Cold, moxibustion is applied to the above points in accordance with patient's conditions; for the case due to Phlegm-Heat, add Fenglong (ST 40) to the prescription; and for the case with severe dyspnea, add Tiantu (RN 22) and Dingchuan (EX-B1).

② The Deficiency syndrome:

Prescription: Feishu (BL 13), Shenshu (BL 23), Gaohuang (BL 43), Qihai (RN 6), Taiyuan (LU 9), Zusanli (ST 36) and Taixi (KI 3).

Manipulation: The above points are treated with reducing method by using filiform needles. Moxibustion is applied in accordance with patient's conditions.

(3) Other therapies:

① Scalp acupuncture: Lateral Line 1 of the Forehead (MS 2) is selected to be punctured with intermittent manipulations of the needle and the needle should be retained for 15 minutes.

② Auricular acupuncture: Select Pingchuan (EP-E7), Adrenal Gland (EP-B 8), Lung (EP-O2), Shenmen (EP-I1) to be needled with manipulations of moderate or strong stimulation. Retain the needles for 20-30 minutes. This is applicable at the attack stage of asthma.

4. Hypertension

Hypertension is a chronic disease marked by persistent elevation of the arterial blood pressure caused by disturbance of the regulatory function of the central nerve system and the endocrine system. Clinically, it is usually diagnosed as long as the blood pressure is over or equal to 21. 3/12kPa in adults. Clinically, it is manifetsed as headache, dizziness, palpitation and blurred vision. In the later stage of the disease, it may involve such important visceral organs as the heart, the brain and the kidney. In TCM, it is called "dizzines" or "headache'.

(1) Syndrome identification:

① Liver Yang rising syndrome: Distending pain of head and eyes, irritability, red face and eyes, bitter taste in the mouth and hyponchondriac pain, constipation, red tongue with little coating or with thin, yellow coating and a wiry pulse.

② Accumulation of Phlegm-Dampness in the Middle-Jiao syndrome: Heaviness of head, headache, vexation, nausea, diarrhea, epigastric fullness, enlarged tongue with white and greasy or white, greasy and thick coating, and a wiry and slippery pulse.

③ Deficiency of Qi and Blood syndrome: Dizziness, aggravated by activity and induced by strain, lassitude, pale and puffy face, palpitation, insomnia, pale tongue, and a fine and weak pulse.

(2) Therapeutic methods:

① Liver Yang rising syndrome:

Prescription: Fengchi (GB 20), Ganshu (BL 18), Shenshu (BL 23), Xingjian (LR 2) and Xiaxi (GL 43).

Manipulation: Puncture with filiform needles by using reducing method.

② Accumulation of Phlegm-Dampness in the Middle-Jiao syndrome:

Prescription: Fenglong (ST 40), Zhongwan (RN 12), Neiguan (PC 6), Jiexi (ST 41) and Touwei (ST 8).

Manipulation: Puncture with filiform needle by adopting uniform reinforcing and reducing method. Moxibustion is applicable.

③ Deficiency of Qi and Blood syndrome:

Prescription: Pishu (BL 20), Zusanli (ST 36), Qihai (RN 6) and Baihui (DU 20).

Manipulation: Puncture with filiform needle by adopting reinforcing method. Moxibustion is applicable.

(3) Other therapy:

Auricular acupuncture: Select Kidney (EP-N4), Liver (EP-N9), Groove for Lowering Blood Pressure (EP-Z1), Shenmen (EP-I1), Endocrine (EP-D1) and Occiput (EP-E5) to be treated with moderate or strong stimulation, 2-3 points each time. Retain the needles for 20-30 minutes in which the needles are manipulated intermittently.

5. Coronary atherosclerotic cardiopathy

This is one kind of heart disease marked by myocardial ischemia and anoxia caused by obstruction of the coronary artery following atherosclerosis of the coronary artery, which is usually manifested as an oppressed feeling in the precardiac region, angina pectoris, accompanied with palpitation and short breath. These symptoms often occur suddenly after violent exercise, emotional stress or exposure to cold, and may be accompanied by cold limbs, perspiration, or even shock and cardiac failure in severe cases. It mostly affects the population over 40 years old, especially the mental workers, and males are more frequently affected than females. In TCM, it is called "chest Bi syndrome" or "true Heart pain".

(1) Syndrome idetification:

① Obstruction of chest Yang syndrome: Chest fullness, shortness of breath, lethargy, lying with limbs huddled up, pale complexion, pale tongue with whitish coating and a wiry, slippery or a wiry, fine pulse.

② Stagnation of Qi and Blood Stasis syndrome: Paroxismal stabbling pain in the precardiac region or the retrosternal region, which radiates to shoulder and back, chest fullness, shortness of breath, or cold limbs, perspiration in sever cases, purplish dark tongue and a deep, uneven or knotted and intermittent pulse.

③ Deficiency of both the Heart and the Spleen syndrome: Oppressed feeling in the precardiac region, lassitude, insomnia, poor appetite, loose stools, pale tongue with whitish coating, a soft weak or a knotted and intermittent pulse.

④ Sudden collapse of the Heart Yang syndrome: Sharp pain in the precardiac region, which is persistent or attacks repeatedly, pal-

139

pitation, dyspnea, cyanotic lips, profuse cold perspiration, cold limbs, coma and a feeble and indistinct pulse.

(2) Therapeutic methods:

① Obstruction of chest Yang syndrome:

Prescription: Zusanli (ST 36), Fenglong (ST 40), Pishu (BL 20), Sanyinjiao (SP 6), Shanzhong (RN 17) and Guanyuan (RN 4).

Manipulation: Shanzhong (RN 17) and Guanyuan (RN 4) are treated by moxibustion with moxa roll; other points are treated by filiform needles with uniform reinforcing and reducing method.

② Stagnation of Qi and Blood Stasis syndrome:

Prescription: Taichong (LR 3), Qimen (LR 4), Xinshu (BL 15), Jueyinshu (BL 14), Neiguan (PC 6) and Tongli (HT 5).

Manipulation: Puncture with filiform needles by adopting reducing method.

③ Deficiency of both the Heart and the Spleen syndrome:

Prescription: Neiguan (PC 6), Xinshu (BL 15), Zusanli (ST 36), Sanyinjiao (SP 6).

Manipulation: Puncture with filiform needles by adopting reinforcing method.

④ Sudden collapse of the Heart Yang syndrome:

Prescription: Baihui (DU 20), Shuigou (DU 26), Guanyuan (RN 4) and Qihai (RN 6).

Manipulation: Guanyuan (RN 4) and Qihai (RN 6) are treated by moxibustion with moxa roll or ginger. Shuigou (DU 26) is treated by using filiform needle with reducing method. Baihui (DU 20) is treated by using filiform needle with uniform reinforcing and reducing method. Needles should be retained until the main symptoms are relieved.

6. Acute gastritis

Acute gastritis is an acute inflammation of the gastric mucous membrane of various causes. Clinically the simple gastritis is mostly seen. And, it usually has a sudden onset, manifested as discomfort or pain in the upper abdomen, anorexia, nausea and vomiting. It often produces diarrhea with watery stools as a result of enteritis being complicated. In TCM, it is called "vomiting" or "epigastric pain".

(1) Syndrome identification:

① The Cold-Dampness syndrome: Abdominal pain, which is relieved by warming, borborygmus, diarrhea with loose stools or even watery stools, thin and whitish tongue coating and a soft and moderate pulse.

② The Dampness-Heat syndrome: Abdominal pain, fulminant diarrhea with black or brown stools, burning sensation in the anus, scanty and dary urine, restlessness, thirst, yellow greasy tongue coating, a soft and rapid or a slippery rapid pulse.

③ The food stagnancy syndrome: This usually has a history of excessive eating or drinking, marked by abdominal pain, borborygmus, diarrhea with fetid stools containing the indigested food after which the abdominal pain is relieved, vomiting with a fetid and sour odour, abdominal fullness, anorexia, thick and greasy tongue coating and a slippery pulse.

(2) Therapeutic methods:

① The Cold-Dampness syndrome:

Prescription: Neiguan (PC 6), Zhongwan (RN 12), Zusanli (St 36).

Manipulation: Zusanli (ST 36) is treated with reinforcing method by using a filiform needle. Other points are treated with reducing method by adopting the filiform needles.

② The Dampness-Heat syndrome:

Prescription: The same as the prescription for the Cold-Dampness syndrome.

Manipulation: Puncture with filiform needles and reducing method.

③ The food stagnancy syndrome:

Prescription: Xiawan (RN 10), Xuanji (RN 21), Zusanli (St 36) and Fujie (SP 14).

Manipulation: Puncture by using filiform needles with reducing method.

(3) Other therapy:

141

Moxibustion therapy: Moxibust the point of the junction of the white and red skin below the tip of the external malleolus with warming moxibustion for 10-15 minutes, 2-3 times a day.

7. Chronic gastritis

Chronic gastritis is a chronic non-specific inflammation of the gastric mucous membrane of varying causes, which is related to immunological factors, regurgitation of the duodenal fluid, delayed acute gastritis, or infections. Clinically, it is manifested as indigestion, burning pain, dull pain or stabbing pain in the upper abdomen, anorexia, nausea, vomiting, acid regurgitation, eructation or even tarry stool. In TCM, it is called "epigastric pain".

(1) Syndrome identification:

① Incoordination between the Liver and the Stomach syndrome: Distending pain in the epigastric region which is migratory and radiates to the bilateral costal regions, poor appetite, eructation, belching, sour and bitter tastes in the mouth, difficulty in defecation, induced by emotional changes, thin and whitish tongue coating and a wiry pulse.

② Deficiency-Cold of the Spleen and Stomach syndrome: Dull pain in the epigastric region, vomiting of clear fluid, desire for warmth and pressure, relieved by warmth, listlessness, poor appetite, loose stools, relatively cold limb, pale tongue with white and greasy coating, and a weak pulse.

③ Deficiency of the Stomach Yin syndrome: Burning pain in the epigastric region, dry mouth and throat, anorexia, gastric discomfort, red tongue with little fluid, a fine and rapid pulse.

(2) Therapeutic methods:

① Incoordination between the Liver and the Stomach syndrome:

Prescription: Neiguan (PC 6), Zhongwan (RN 12), Zusanli (ST 36), Yanglingquan (GB 34), Taichong (LR 3).

Manipulation: Puncture by using filiform needles with reducing method.

② Deficiency-Cold of the Spleen and the Stomach syndrome:

Prescription: Neiguan (PC 6), Zhongwan (RN 12), Zusanli (St 36), Pishu (BL 20) and Weishu (BL 21).

Manipulation: Puncture with reinforcing method by using filiform needles.

③ Deficiency of the Stomach Yin syndrome:

Prescription: Zusanli (St 36), Zhongwan (RN 12), Neiting (ST 44) and Taixi (KI 3).

Manipulation: Puncture with reinforcing method by using filiform needles.

(3) Other therapy:

Auricular acupuncture: Select Spleen (EP-N10), Stomach (EP-M4), Shenmen (EP-I1), Sympathetic (EP-H1), Subcortex (EP-E10) to be needled, 2-3 points each time with needle retained for 15-30 minutes. Needle-embedding therapy is applicable.

8. Gastroptosis

Gastroptosis indicates entering of the great curvature of the stomach into the pelvic cavity or the lowest point of the lesser curvature being lower than the line connecting the two illiac spines in a standing position. It is one kind of prolapse of the visceral organs, and is mostly caused by decrease of the tension of the abdominal wall, relaxation or weakness of the gastrophrenic ligament, the hepatogastric ligament or the abdominal muscles. Clinically, it is marked by a lowering down sensation in the abdomen, poor appetite, which is more severe after eating, dull pain in the upper abdomen, eructation, acid regurgitation, alternate occurrence of scanty stools, diarrhea and constipation. In TCM, it is called "abdominal distension", "epigastric pain" or "gastric discomfort".

(1) Syndrome identification:

Sinking of the Middle-Jiao Qi syndrome: Dull pain or lowering down sensation in the epigastric region, which is more severe after eating and relieved by pressure, desire for hot food or drinks, anorexia, lassitude, lustreless face, pale tongue with whitish coating, and a deep, fine and weak pulse.

(2) Therapeutic method:

Prescription: Zhongwan (RN 12), Zusanli (ST 36), Weishang (2 cun above the umbilicus, 4 cun lateral to the anterior midline), Baihui (DU 20).

143

Manipulation: Puncture by using filiform needles with reinforcing method. Moxibustion can be applied to Baihui (DU 20). And, Weishang and Zhongwan (RN 12) are treated by inserting the needle from Weishang to allow the needle to penetrate to Zhongwan (RN 12) with reinforcing method by twisting and rotating the needle until a feeling of the stomach being lifted is felt.

(3) Other therapy:

Auricular acupuncture therapy: Select Spleen (Ep-N10), Stomach (Ep-M4), Liver (N9), Shenmen (EP-I1) to treat the disease with moderate stimulation. The needles should be retained for 1 hour and the treatment is performed once every other day.

9. Peptic ulcer

This is a chronic ulcer appearing mainly in the stomach and the duodenal bulb or in the lower portion of the esophagus, the tissues around the gastrojujunal opening and the Meckel's diverticulum. In most cases, its formation is related to the digestive function of the gastric acid and the pepsin. This disease is usually seen in young or middle aged people, with regular epigastric pain, eructation, acid regurgitation, nausea, vomiting, burning sensation in the stomach, or even hematemesis and hemafecia as its main manifestations. In TCM, it is called "epigastric pain".

(1) Syndrome identification:

① Attack of pathogenic Cold on the Stomach syndrome: Sudden sharp pain in the epigastric region, dislike cold and desire for warmth, no thrist, desire for hot drinks, thin and whitish tongue coating, and a wiry tense pulse.

② Attack of the Stomach by the Liver Qi syndrome: Distending pain in the eigastric region, which radiates to the costal regions, frequent eructation, difficult defecation, which are aggravated by emotional depression, or irritability, severe gastric pain, acid regurgitation, red tonge with yellow coating, and a wiry or rapid pulse.

③ Deficiency-Cold of the Spleen and Stomach syndrome: Dull pain in the epigastric region which can be relieved by pressure and warmth and is more severe at an empty stomach, relieved or aggravated by eating, vomiting of watery fluid, listlessness, lassitude,

144

loose stools, cold limbs, pale tongue with whitish coating, and a weak or slow pulse.

④ Blood Stasis syndrome: Stabbling pain in the epigastric region, which is fixed and aggravated by pressure, hematemesis, hamefecia, dark purplish tongue and a hesitant pulse.

(2) Therapeutic methods:

① Attack of pathogenic Cold on the Stomach syndrome:

Prescription: Zusanli (ST 36), Zhongwan (RN 12), Weishu (BL 21).

Manipulation: Zusanli (ST 36) is treated by using a filiform needle with reducing method. Other points are treated by adopting moxibustion with ginger until 7-10 moxa cones are burnt.

② Attack of the Stomach by Liver Qi syndrome:

Prescription: Liangmen (ST 21), Qimen (LR 14), Taichong (LR 3), Neiguan (PC 6), Zusanli (St 36).

Manipulation: Puncture by adopting filiform needles with reducing method.

③ Deficiency-Cold of the Spleen and the Stomach syndrome:

Prescription: Pishu (BL 20), Weishu (BL 21), Zhongwan (RN 12), Zhangmen (LR 13).

Manipulation: Puncture by using filiform needles with reinforcing method. Moxibustion is applied after acupuncture.

④ Blood Stasis syndrome:

Prescription: Geshu (BL 17), Neiguan (PC 6), Xuehai (SP 10), Gongsun (SP 4).

Manipulation: Puncture by using filiform needles with uniform reinforcing and reducing method.

(3) Other therapy:

Auricular acupuncture: Select Stomach (EP-M4), Duodenum (EP-M5), Mouth (EP-M1), Sympathetic (EP-H1) and Subcortex (EP-E20) to be needled with moderate stimulation. The treatment is performed once every day for the disease at the acute stage, and once every other day for the diseases at the remission stage.

10. Gastrointestinal neurosism

This is a general term for a group of syndromes of the stomach

145

and the intestines. It is mostly caused by emotional stimuli and is marked by disturbance of the peristalsis of the gastrointestinal tract. Pathologically, no organic disease is found and it doesn't include the functional disturbance of the gastrointestinal tract secondary to diseases of other systems. Clinically, it is manifested as the symptoms concerning with the gastrointestinal tract, such as insomnia, anxiety, forgetfulness, headache, and nervousness. This disease mostly affects the young and the middle aged, and in TCM, it is called "gastric pain" or "mental depression".

(1) Syndrome identification:

① Attack of the Stomach by the Liver Qi syndrome: Distension in the epigastric region which radiates to the costal region and is migratory, frequent eructation which is aggravated by emotional depression, thin and whitish coating and a wiry pulse.

② Incoordination between the Liver and the Spleen syndrome: Abdominal distension, loose stools, poor appetite, epigastric fullness after eating, or constipation, which occur or are aggravated by emotional stress or depression, pale tongue with whitish coating and a wiry pulse.

(2) Therapeutic methods:

① Attack of the Stomach by the Liver Qi syndrome:

Prescription: Yanglingquan (GB 34), Zhongwan (RN 12), Liangqiu (ST 34), Shenmen (H 7) and Neiguan (PC 6).

Manipulation: Puncture by using filiform needles with reducing method.

② Incoordination between the Liver and the Spleen syndrome:

Prescription: Zusanli (ST 36), Taichong (LR 3), Tianshu (ST 25), Sanyinjiao (SP 6), Shangjuxu (ST 37).

Manipulation: Puncture by adopting filiform needles with reinforcing method except Taichong (LR 3) which is treated with reducing method.

(3) Other therapy:

Auricular acupuncture: Select Liver (EP-N9), Spleen (EP-N10), Sympathetic (EP-H1), Shenmen (EP-I1) and Subcortex (EP-E10) to be treated with moderate or strong timulation. The needles are

146

retained for 15-20 minutes and the treatment is done once daily.

11. Infection of the biliary tract and cholelithasis

Infection of the biliary tract includes the acute and chronic chole-cystitis and infection of the biliary duct. Cholelithiasis includes cholecystolithiasis, coledocholithiasis and hepatolith. These diseases mainly affect the young people and woman is more frequently affected than man. The infection of the biliary tract is usually caused by biliary obstruction, cholestasis and bacterial infection of the biliary tract; while the cholelithiasis is mostly caused by metabolic disturbance of the bilirubin and cholesterol or foreign bodies in the biliary tract. These two diseases often coexist and have a cause-result relationship. The infection of the biliary tract is clinically manifested by chills, high fever, pain in the right upper abdomen, which is aggravated progressively, jaundice, or accompanied with indigestion. In chronic case, it may present dull pain or stabbing pain in the right upper abdomen, which is more severe after eating fatty food. The cholelithiaisis may cause colic, obstructive jaundice or the symptoms of infection of the biliary tract. In TCM, it is called "hypochondrium" or "jaundice".

(1) Syndrome identification:

① Stagnation of Qi syndrome: Distending pain in the right upper abdomen, which radiates to the shoulder and back, accompanied with bitter taste in the mouth, dry throat, poor appetite, abdominal distension, absence of jaundice, thin whitish or yellowish tongue coating, and a wiry tense pulse.

② Dampness-Heat syndrome: Colicky pain in the costal region and epigastric region, which is aggravated paroxismally and by pressure, accompanied with poor appetite, bitter taste in the mouth, chills, high fever, nausea, vomiting, constipation, dark urine, or accompanied by jaundice, red tongue with yellow greasy coating, and a wiry, slippery and rapid pulse.

③ Septicemia syndrome: Persistent severe pain in the costal and epigastric region, which radiates to the shoulder and back, rigidity of the abdominal muscles with ternderness, jaundice, thirst, scanty urine, constipation, or even coma, delirium, red or deep red tongue

147

with yellow and rough coating, and a wiry slippery and rapid or a fine and rapid pulse.

(2) Therapeutic method:

Prescription: Danshu (BL 19), Ganshu (BL 18), Riyue (GB 24), Qimen (LR 14), Yanglingquan (GB 34), Dannangxue (EX-LE6), Taichong (LR 3).

Manipulation: Puncture by adopting filiform needles with strong reducing method. For cases due to Qi stagnation, add Xingjian (LR 2); for cases due to Damp-Heat, add Zusanli (ST 36) and Yinlingquan (SP 9); for cases with septicemia, add Shuigou (DU 26), Dazhui (DU 14), Neiguan (PC 6) and Zulinqi (GB 41); for cases with colicky pain, add Hegu (LI 4) and Ximen (PC 4); and for cases with jaundice, add Zhiyin (DU 9).

(3) Other therapies:

① Electric acupuncture: 3 or 4 of the following points, Danshu (BL 19), Qimen (LR 4), Riyue (GB 24), Zhongwan (RN 12), Yanglingquan (GB 34), Liangmen (ST 21), Taichong (LR 3), Dannang (EX-LE6), are selected each time. The points are from both the local area and the remote area. When the feeling of gaining Qi occurs, connect the needles with the electric acupuncture instrument. Dannangxue (BL 19) and Zhongwan (RN 12) are connected with the cathod; while Taichong (LR 3), Yanglingquan (GB 34), Dannang (EX-LE6) are connected with anode. Treat the disease with adjustable wave by increasing the intensity from weak to strong until patient cannot bear. 30 minutes each time, 1-3 times daily.

② Auricular acupuncture: Select 2-4 points of Pancreas (EP-N6), Liver (EP-N9), Duodenum (EP-M5), Shenmen (EP-I1), Sympathetic (EP-H1) and Triple-Jiao (EP-O5) each time to be treated with strong stimulation. The needles are retained 30-60 minutes with intermittent manipulations of the needles, once daily.

12. Ulcerous colitis

Ulcerous colitis is a non-specific inflammatory disease of the retum and colon with unknown reasons, which is mainly manifested as diarrhea with stools containing mucous fluid or blood, abdominal pain and tenesmus in the clinic. It may affect the population of any age, but it is mostly seen in the young and the middle aged people. At present, it is generally believed that occurrence of the disease is related to abnormality of the immunological function, allergic reaction and inheritary constitution. In TCM, it is called "diarrhea".

(1) Syndrome identification:

① Weakness of the Spleen and the Stomach syndrome: Frequent occurrence of loose stools or diarrhea with indigested food, distension in the epigastric region and abdomen, increase of the frequency of defecation after eating less fatty food, sallow complexion, lassitude, pale tongue with whitish coating, and a fine and weak pulse.

② Deficiency of both the Spleen Yang and the Kidney Yang syndrome: Abdominal pain at dawn followed by borborygmus and diarrhea after which the abdominal pain is relieved, accompanied with aversion to cold, cold limbs, soreness and weakness of the loins and knees, abdominal fullness, poor appetite, pale tongue with whitish coating, and a deep, fine pulse.

(2) Therapeutic methods:

① Weakness of the Spleen and the Stomach syndrome:

Prescription: Zhongwan (RN 12), Tianshu (ST 25), Zusanli (ST 36), Shangjuxu (ST 37), Yinlingquan (SP 9) and Sanyinjiao (SP 6).

Manipulation: Puncture by using filiform needles with reinforcing method. Moxibustion may be applied concurrently.

② Deficiency of both the Spleen Yang and the Kidney Yang syndrome:

Prescription: Zhongwan (RN 12), Pishu (BL 20), Zhangmen (LR 13), Tainshu (ST 25), and Zusanli (ST 36).

Manipulation: Puncture with reinforcing method by using filiform needles. Moxibustion may be applied simultaneously.

(3) Other therapy:

Auricular acupuncture: Select Small Intestine (EP-M6), Large Intestine (EP-M8), Stomach (EP-M4), Spleen (EP-N10), Sympathetic (EP-H1), Shenmen (EP-I1) and Lower Portion of Rectum (EP-K15) to be needled with moderate stimulation. The needles are retained for 10-20 minutes, and the treatment is performed once daily.

13. Habitual constipation

This is a disease marked by difficulty in defecation, dry stools or the interval of two defecations being over 48 hours with discomfort, which is usually caused by mental disorders, disorders of the nerves, decrease of the motive force for defecation, weakening of the stress ability of the intestinal mucous membrane, or disappearance of the defecation reflex. In TCM, it is called "inhibition of the Spleen", or "constipation".

(1) Syndrome identification:

① The Excess syndrome: Reduce of frequency of defectaion, one bowel movement every 3-5 days or even longer than that, dry stools which is difficult to be discharged though patient works hard. If it is caused by accumulation of Heat, there is fever, severe thirst, fetid odour in the mouth, desire for cold drinks, yellow and dry tongue coating, and a slippery and forceful pulse; if it is caused by stagnation of Qi, there is distending pain in the costal region and abdomen, eructation, poor appetite, thin and greasy tongue coating and a wiry pulse.

② The Deficiency syndrome: In the cases caused by Qi deficiency, there is pale and puffy face, lustreless nails and lips, dizziness, palpitation, listlessness, feeble voice, pale tongue with thin whitish coating and a feeble and fine pulse. In the cases due to accumulation of Yin Cold, there is cold pain in the abdomen, desire for hotness and dislike of cold, pale tongue with whitish coating and a deep slow pulse.

(1) Therapeutic methods:

① The Excess syndrome:

Prescription: Dachangshu (BL 25), Tianshu (ST 25), Zhigou (SJ 6), Shangjuxu (ST 37) and Hegu (LI 4).

Manipulation: Puncture with reducing method by using filiform needles.

② The Deficiency syndrome:

Prescription: Dachangshu (BL 25), Tianshu (ST 25), Zusanli (ST 36), Sanyinjiao (SP 6) and Pishu (BL 20).

150

Manipulation: Puncture with reinforcing method by adopting fili-form needles. For cases due to Qi Deficiency, add Qihai (RN 6); for cases with depletion of Body Fluid, add Taixi (KI 3) and Fuliu (KI 7); and for cases due to accumulation of Cold, add Shenque (RN 8) and Guanyuan (RN 4) to be treated with moxibustion.

(3) Other therapy:

Electric acupuncture: Select Daheng (SP 15), Xiajuxu (ST 39), Shimen (RN 5) and Zhigou (SJ 6) to be treated with sparse-intense waves with the needle retained for 10-20 minutes. The treatment is performed once a day or once every other day, and the above 4 points are adopted alternately.

14. Pyelonephritis

Pyeonephritis is an inflammation of the mucous membrane of the pelvis of the kidney and the renal calyx, as well as the renal tubules and the interstitia of the kidney caused by various kinds of pathogenic organisms, especially the ascending inflammation of bac-teria. It mostly affects the female with lumbago and frequent, ur-gent and painful urination as its main manifestations. Clinically, it can be classified as two types, the acute and the chronic. The for-mer may be accompanied with fever, chills, general discomfort and appetite; and the latter, which often develops from the former, is often accompanied with lasstidue, lower fever and increase of night urination. In TCM, it is called "stranguria".

(1) Syndrome identification:

① Damp-Heat in the Bladder syndrome: Urgent dark and hot urine with a burning sensation accopmanied with fever, yellow greasy tongue coating and a slippery rapid pulse.

② Yin Deficiency with pathogen lingering syndrome: Burning sensation or pain during urination, thirst with a desire for drinking, feverish sensation over the palms and soles, obvious soreness of loins, red tongue with little coating and a fine and rapid pulse.

③ Deficiency of both the Spleen Yang and the Kidney Yang syn-drome: Difficult and painful urination with dribbling, a lowering sensation in the loins or sacral region, dull pain in the lumbar re-gion, increase of nocturnal urination, which are often induced or ag-

151

gravated by physical strain or sexual intercourse, pale tongue with a thin and whitish coating and a deep and fine pulse.

(2) Therapeutic methods:

① Damp-Heat in the Bladder syndrome:

Prescription: Pangguangshu (BL 28), Zhongji (RN 3), Yinlingquan (SP 9) and Weizhong (BL 40).

Manipulation: Puncture with reducing method by adopting filiform needles.

② Yin Deficiency with pathogen lingering syndrome:

Prescription: Shenshu (BL 23), Pangguangshu (BL 28), Zhongji (RN 3), Taixi (KI 3), Zhaohai (KI 6) and Sanyinjiao (SP 6).

Manipulation: Puncture by using filiform needles with reducing method first followed by reinforcing method in Shenshu (BL 23), reinforcing method in Taixi (KI 3), Zhaohai (KI 6) and Sanyinjiao (SP 6) and uniform reinfocing and reducing method in Pangguangshu (BL 28) and Zhongji (RN 3).

③ Deficiency of both the Spleen Yang and the Kidney Yang syndrome:

Prescription: Shenshu (BL 23), Pishu (BL 20), Zhongji (RN 3), Zusanli (ST 36) and Qihai (RN 6).

Manipulation: Puncture by using filiform needle with reinforcing method.

(3) Other therapy:

Auricular acupuncture: Select Kidney (EP-N 4), Spleen (EP-N 10), Bladder (EP-N 1), Triple-Jiao (EP-O 5), Endocrine (EP-D 1), Adrenal gland (EP-B 8), Urethra (EP-K 14) to be treated with moderate stimulation, 3-5 points are chosen each time with the needles retained for 20-30 minutes, once every 2 days.

15. Stone in urinary system

This is a general term for stones in different parts of the urinary system including the kidney, the ureter, bladder and the urethra, which is marked by the local damage, obstruction and inflammation of the urinary system following the formation of the stone. It is usually caused by retention of urine arising from stenosis of obstruction of the urinary system, obstruction or foreign bodies in the urinary

152

system. Its clinical manifestations vary with the different portions of the urinary system affected. Stone in the kidney or the ureter often causes colic of the kidney and hematuria; that in the bladder often causes difficulty in discharging urine, terminal hematuria and pain during urination; and that or the urethra often causes difficulty in discharging urine or even retention of urine. In most cases, the stones are complicated by infection of different parts of the urinary stsem, and the disease is mainly seen in males. In TCM, it is called "stranguria with bloody urine" and "stranguria with stone".

(1) Syndrome identification:

① Dampness-Heat in the Lower-Jiao syndrome: Colicky pain in the loins and abdomen, difficult, dribbling and painful urination, sudden blockage of the urine discharge, or hematuria with sands or stone, or vexation, bitter taste in the mouth, constipation, yellow and greasy tongue coating, and a wiry, slippery or a slippery rapid pulse.

② Stagnation of Qi and Blood Stasis syndrome: Dull pain or colicky pain in the loins and abdomen, or even hematuria, sudden blockage of the urine discharge, purplish tongue which may be dotted with ecchymosis with a thin coating, and a wiry tense pulse.

③ Kidney Deficiency syndrome: No strength to discharge urine or painful urination, soreness in the loins and knees, or dizziness, tinnitus, feverish sensation over the palms, soles and chest, night sweat, red tongue with little coating and a fine rapid pulse, or pale and puffy complexion, aversion to cold, cold limbs, pale tongue with whitish coating, and deep fine pulse.

(2) Therapeutic methods:

① Dampness-Heat in the Lower-Jiao syndrome:

Prescription: Shenshu (BL 23), Yinlingquan (SP 9), Weiyang (BL 39), Sanyinjiao (SP 6) and Jingmen (GB 25).

Manipulation: Puncture by using filiform needles with reducing method.

② Stagnation of Qi and Blood Stasis syndrome:

Prescription: Shenshu (BL 23), Jingmen (GB 25), Qihai (RN 6), Ququan (LR 8), Weizhong (BL 40).

Manipulation: Puncture by using filiform needles, with reinforcing method in Shenshu (BL 23) and Jingmen (GB 25) and reducing method in Qihai (RN 6), Ququan (LR 8) and Weizhong (BL 40).

③ Kidney Deficiency syndrome:

Prescription: Shenshu (BL 23), Pangguangshu (BL 28), Sanyinjiao (SP 6) and Yinlingquan (SP 9).

Manipulation: Puncture by adopting filiform needles with reinforcing method. In the case of Deficiency of the Kidney Yang, add moxibustion on Mingmen (DU 4) and Guanyuan (RN 4) additionally; and in the case of Kidney Yin Deficiency, add Zhongji (RN 3) and Taixi (KI 3) to be punctured by using filiform needles with reinforcing method.

(3) Other therapy:

Electric acupuncture: Select Shenshu (BL 23) and Sanyinjiao (SP 6) to be treated with strong stimulation of high frequency. The needles are retained for 5-10 minutes.

16. Retention of urine

Retention of urine indicates excessive filling of urine in bladder and failure of the urine to be discharged, which is mostly caused by diseases of the central urinary system, injury to nerves, pain in the urethra, prostate gland or around the anus, hysterica, stenosis or stone of the urethra, hypertrophy of the prostate gland, and peripheral abscess of the urethra. Clinically it is classfied as two types: the acute and the chronic, and in TCM, it is called "uroschesis".

(1) Syndrome identification:

① Deficiency of the Kidney Qi syndrome: Dribbling of urine, no enough power to discharge urine, pale and puffy face, soreness and weakness of the loins and knees, pale tongue, deep fine pulse which is also weak in the Chi portion.

② Downward flow of Dampness-Heat syndrome: Scanty and dark urine with a hot sensation, or even failure of the urine to be discharged, distension in the lower abdomen, thirst, red tongue with yellow coating, and a rapid pulse.

③ Traumatic injury: Oliguria, failure to discharge urine, fullness and distension in the lower abdomen, with a history of traumatic injury or surgical operation.

(2) Therapeutic methods:

① Deficiency of the Kidney Qi syndrome:

Prescription: Yingu (KI 10), Shenshu (KI 23), Sanjiaoshu (BL 22), Qihai (RN 6) and Weiyang (BL 39).

Manipulation: Puncture by using filiform needles with reinforcing method.

② Downward flow of Dampness-Heat syndrome:

Prescription: Sanyinjiao (SP 6), Yinlingquan (SP 9), Pangguangshu (BL 28) and Zhongji (RN 3).

Manipulation: Puncture by using filiform needles with reducing method.

③ Traumatic injury:

Prescription: Zhongji (RN 3) and Sanyinjiao (SP 6).

Manipulation: Puncture by using filiform needles with uniform reinforcing and reducing method.

(3) Other therapy:

Scalp acupunture: Select Lateral Line 3 of Forehead (MS4) to be punctured 1. 5 cun with a 1. 5 cun long filiform needle subcutaneously and obliquely toward the back of neck by adopting the reducing method, 20 minutes each time, once daily.

17. Leukopenia

Leukopenia is a disease marked by constant reduce of the total amount of the peripheral leukocytes, which is less than 4000/ mm^3, with decrease of the granulocytes as its main feature. This disease is divided into two types: That caused by unknown reasons and that secondary to other diseases. The former has a slow onset and may not present special symptoms, and in a few cases, it is revealed when the patients receive physical examination; while the latter are often related to administration of drugs, infection, exposure to radioactive rays or some other diseases. Clinically, this disease is characterized by dizziness, lassitude, soreness and weakness of the limbs, poor appetite, low fever, etc. , and in TCM it is called "consumptive disease".

(1) Syndrome identification:

① Deficiency of the Spleen Qi syndrome: Dizziness, lassitude, poor appetite, listlessness, loose stools, sallow complexion, pale tongue with a thin and whitish coating, and a soft and weak pulse.

② Kidney Deficiency syndrome: Dizziness, vertigo, soreness and weakness of the loins and knees, dysuria, or aversion to cold, cold limbs, pain with a cold feeling in the lower abdomen, pale tongue, whitish coating with much fluids, and a fine and rapid pulse.

(2) Therapeutic method:

Prescription: Zusanli (ST 36), Sanyinjiao (SP 6), Geshu (BL 17), Xuehai (SP 10).

Manipulation: Puncture by adopting filiform needles with reinforcing method. In the case of Deficiency of the Spleen Qi, add Pishu (BL 20); in the case of Deficiency of the Kidney Yang, add Shenshu (BL 23) and Guanyuan (RN 4); and in the case of Deficiency of the Kidney Yin, add Shenshu (BL 23) and Taixi (KI 3).

(3) Other therapy:

Moxibustion: Select Dazhui (DU 14), Mingmen (DU 4) and Zusanli (ST 36) to be moxibusted with moxa cone, 3 *Zhuang* each time, once daily.

18. Obesity

When a person takes in more heat energy then that he consumes, the excessive heat will store in the form of fat in the body, causing a body weight which is 20% more than the standard weight or a result of the index (kg) of the body weight divided by the height of body (M^2) being more than 24. (in foreign countries, the result should be 27 in male and 25 in female in normal conditions.) This condition is referred to as obesity, which is of two types: The simple obesity and the secondary obesity. It is generally believed that this disease is related to defect of inheridity, nervous system, mental activities and the endocrine system, and it is clinically manifested by laziness, lethargy, listlessness, lassitude, hyperrexia, polyhidrosis, aversion to hot, chest stuffiness and palpitation.

(1) Syndrome identification:

① Spleen Deficiency with exuberance of Dampness syndrome: Over weight, epigastric and abdominal fullness, flat taste in the mouth, anorexia, heaviness of the head and body, feeble voice, disinclination to talk, pale tongue with white and greasy coating, and a soft and weak pulse.

② Deficiency of both the Spleen and the Kidney syndrome: Over weight, aversion to cold, cold limbs, lethargy, listlessness, lassitude, soreness and weakness of the loins and knees, hyposexualism, pale tongue with thin and whitish coating, and fine, soft and feeble pulse.

(2) Therapeutic methods:

① Spleen Deficiency with exuberance of Dampness syndrome:

Prescription: Lieque (LU 7), Shaofu (HT 8), Yinlingquan (SP 9), Sanyinjiao (SP 6), Fenglong (ST 40).

Manipulation: Puncture with a filiform needle by adopting the uniform reinforcing and reducing method.

② Deficiency of both the Spleen and the Kidney syndrome:

Prescription: Pishu (BL 20), Shenshu (BL 23), Zusanli (ST 36), Sanyinjiao (SP 6), Daheng (SP 15).

Manipulation: Puncture with a filiform needle by adopting reinforcing method.

(3) Other therapy:

Auricular acupuncture: Select Spleen (EP-N 10), Stomach (EP-M4), Mouth (EP-M1), Esophagus (EP-M2), Adrenal Gland (EP-B8) and Endocrine (EP-D1) to be needled with strong stimulation, 3-5 points each time with the needles retaining 20-30 minutes, once every other day, or to be treated with needle-embedding.

19. Hyperlipidemia and hyperlipoproteinemia

That the concentration of blood lipid in plasma is higher than the maximal amount of a normal condition is known as hyperlipidemia; while when the concentration of the lipid proteins in plasma is higher than the maximal amount of the normal one, it is termed hyperlipoproteinemia. The hyperlipdemia is often complicated by hyperlipoproteinemia. The disease can be divided into either the primary or the secondary. The former is unknown in causes and most patients have a family history or an inheritary history; while the latter may be secondary to such diseases as diabetes, pancreatitis or coronary heart disease. In TCM, it is called "dizziness".

(1) Syndrome identification:

① Accumulation of Dampness-Heat in the interior syndrome: Dizziness, vertigo, lassitude, fullness in the epigastric region and abdomen, heaviness of the limbs, chest stuffiness, poor appetite, red and enlarged tongue with teethmarks on its border, greasy tongue coating, and a feeble, large and slippery pulse.

② Stagnation of Qi and Blood Stasis syndrome: Palpitation, chest stuffiness or even chest pain referring to the costal region, anorexia, abdominal distension, irritability, eructation, disorders of defecation, purple tongue or dotted with ecchymosis, and a wiry or fine and uneven pulse.

(2) Therapeutic methods:

① Accumulation of Dampness-Heat in the interior syndrome:

Prescription: Taibai (SP 3), Zusanli (ST 36), Fenglong (ST 40), Shangjuxu (ST 37).

Manipulation: Puncture by using filiform needles with reducing method on Fenglong (ST 40) and Shangjuxu (ST 37), and with reinforcing methods on other points in this prescription.

② Stagnation of Qi and Blood Stasis syndrome:

Prescription: Yanglingquan (GB 34), Ganshu (BL 18), Geshu (BL 17), and Shanzhong (RN 17).

Manipulation: Puncture by using filiform needles with reducing method in Ganshu (BL 18) and Geshu (BL 17), and with the uniform reinforcing and reducing method on other points in this prescription.

(3) Other therapy:

Electric acupuncture: Select Ququan (LR 8), Neiguan (PC 6), Zusanli (ST 36) and Quchi (LI 11) to be needled. When the feeling of gaining Qi occurs, connect the needles with the electric acupuncture instrument and administer a stimulation that the patient can bear, 15 minutes each time, once every other day.

20. Rheumatoid arthritis

Rheumatoid arthritis is a systemic disease with chronic and symmetrical inflammation of multiple joints as its main pathologic

changes, which is generally believed to be an autoimmunological re
action due to infection, which leads to the disease of joints marked
by synovitis. Swelling, pain or even stiffness, deformity and severe
dysfunction of the joints in the later stage are the common symptoms of the disease. In TCM, it is called "arthralgia syndrome".

(1) Syndrome identification:

① Arthralgia caused by Wind, Cold and Dampness syndrome: Severe arthralgia, aggravated by cold and relieved by heat, numbness
and heaviness of joints, difficulty of the joints in movements, pale
and enlarged tongue with a whitish and greasy tongue coating, and a
wiry slippery pulse.

② Arthralgia caused by Wind, Cold and Heat syndrome: Swelling
and pain of the joints with a hot sensation, aggravated by heat and
relieved by cold, difficulty of the joints in movements, thirst, polyhidrosis, scanty and dark urine, red tongue with a yellow coating,
and a rapid and slippery pulse.

③ Kidney Deficiency and stagnation of pathogenic Cold syndrome: Deformity of the joints, muscular atrophy, dizziness, vertigo, soreness and weakness of the loins and knees, frequent reccur-
rence, purplish dark tongue, and a fine and unevenm pulse.

(2) Therapeutic methods:

① Arthralgia caused by Wind, Cold and Dampness syndrome:

Prescription: Fengmen (BL 12), Yanglingquan (GB 34), Pishu
(BL 20), Shenshu (BL 23), Guanyuan (RN 4).

Manipulation: Puncture by adopting filiform needles, with reducing method on Fengmen (BL 12) and Yanglingquan (GB 34) and reinforcing method on other points in this prescription. Besides, the
disease may also be treated by puncturing the local points of the
joints.

② Arthralgia caused by Wind, Cold and Heat syndrome:

Prescription: Dazhui (DU 14), Quchi (LI 11), Pishu (BL 20),
Yanglingquan (SP 9) and Sanjiaoshu (BL 22).

Manipulation: Puncture by using filiform needles with reducing
method, except Pishu (BL 20) which is treated with reinforcing
method. Besides, the local points of the joints may also be selected

to be treated.

③ Kidney Deficiency and stagnation of pathogenic Cold syndrome:

Prescription: Shenshu (BL 23), Ganshu (BL 18), Pishu (BL 20), Geshu (BL 17), Fenglong (ST 40), and Zusanli (ST 36).

Manipulation: Puncture by using filiform needles with reinforcing method, except for Geshu (BL 17) and Fenglong (ST 40) which are treated with reducing method.

21. Impotence

This is a disease marked by failure of the penis to erect or to become hard enough to carry out the sexual intercourse in sexual life, which is either functional or organic. The functional impotence, more commonly seen than the organic in the clinic, is in relation to emotional states, and is marked by inability of the penis to erect in sexual life but erecting of the penis in onanism or when the urine is filled fully in the bladder during sleep, although the erected penis is not hard enough or the erecting lasts a short time. The organic impotence, however, is usually caused by anatomical reasons, drugs or other diseases, and clinically it is marked by inability of the penis to erect in any conditions. In TCM, it is called "impotence", and it falls into the category of dysfunction of male sexualism.

(1) Syndrome identification:

① Decline of the Kidney Yang syndrome: Failure of the penis to erect, cold and thin sperma, frequent nocturnal urine, dizziness, tiniitus, lassitude, soreness and weakness of the loins and knees, aversion to cold, cold limbs, pale tongue, and a deep, fine and slow pulse.

② Deficiency of both the Heart and the Spleen syndrome: Hyposexuality, failure of the penis to erect hardly, palpitation, liability to be frightened, insomnia, forgetfulness, sallow complexion, shortness of breath, lassitude, abdominal fullness, loose stools, pale tongue with thin and whitish coating, and a deep, weak pulse.

③ Stagnation of the Liver Qi syndrome: Failure of the penis to erect, mental depression, chest fullness, anorexia, frequent sighing, fullness and disconfort in the costal region or in the lower ab-

160

domen, or a feeling of foreign body obstructing in the throat, pale tongue with thin and whitish coating, and a wiry pulse.

④ Dampness-Heat in the Liver and Gallbladder syndrome: Softness of the penis, failure of the penis to erect hardly, wet scrotum, or distending pain in the testis or lower abdomen, dark urine, pain in the penis, or dribbling of urine, bitter taste in the mouth, dry mouth, irritability, soreness and weakness of the lower limbs, red tongue with yellow and sticky tongue coating, and a wiry and rapid pulse.

(2) Therapeutic methods:

① Decline of the Kidney Yang syndrome:

Prescription: Dazhui (DU 14), Mingmen (DU 4), Shanshu (BL 23), Guanyuanshu (BL 26), Sanyinjiao (SP 6).

Manipulation: Puncture by adopting filiform needles with reinforcing method. Moxibustion may be applied simultaneously.

② Deficiency of both the Heart and the Spleen syndrome:

Prescription: Xinshu (BL 15), Neiguan (PC 6), Sanyinjiao (SP 6), Zusanli (ST 36), Guanyuan (RN 4).

Manipulation: Puncture by using filiform needles with reinforcing method, and moxibustion is applied to each of the points after needling.

③ Stagnation of the Liver Qi syndrome:

Prescription: Ganshu (BL 18), Qimen (LR 4), Taichong (LR 3), Qugu (RN 2), Ququan (LR 8).

Manipulation: Puncture by using filiform needles with uniform reinforcing and reducing method.

④ Dampness-Heat in the Liver and Gallbladder syndrome:

Prescription: Ligou (LR 5), Sanyinjiao (SP 6), Taichong (LR 3), Yinlingquan (SP 9), Shenshu (BL 23), Qugu (RN 2).

Manipulation: Puncture by using filiform needles with the reducing method first and then the reinforcing method.

(3) Other therapies:

① Auricular acupuncture: Select Kidney (EP-N4), External Genital (EP-K13), Shenmen (EP-I1) and Subcortex (EP-E10), Endocrine (EP-K13) to be treated with moderate stimulation, 2-3 points each time with the needles retaining 15-30 minutes, once every day or once every other day.

② Electric acupuncture: Select Ciliao (BL 32), Ranggu (KI 2), Guanyuan (RN 4), and Sanyinjiao (SP 6) to be treated alternately with low frequency stimulation, once every other day. The needles should be retained for 10-20 minutes.

Neuropsychopathy

1. Trigeminal neuralgia

This refers to the recurrent, transient and paroxysmal sharp pain appearing in the area where the trigeminal nerve is distributed, which can be divided into the primary and the secondary. The primary trigeminal neuralgia has not a clearly identified cause, while the secondary one is usually caused by stimuli of the inflammation of the eyes, the nose or the teeth, press of the tumour and malnutrition of the nervous system. This disease mostly affects the population aged from 40 to 60, and female are more susceptible to the disease. Clinically it is mainly marked by a sudden sharp pain which gives a feeling of bearing an electric shock, being cut with a knife, teared or scorched. In TCM, it is called "face pain" or "wind of head".

(1) Syndrome identification:

① Obstruction of Wind and Cold syndrome: Paroxysmal sharp pain as if being pricked or cut in one side of the face, which is often aggravated by pressure and affection of cold and relieved by warmth, thin and whitish tongue coating, and floating tense pulse.

② Excess Heat in Yangming channel syndrome: Paroxysmal sharp pain as being burnt or scorched in the face, which is aggravated by exposure to wind or Heat, thirst, fetid odour in the mouth, irritability, constipation, dark urine, yellow tongue coating with little fluid, and a full, large or a slippery and rapid pulse.

③ Hyperactivity of Yang due to Yin Deficiency syndrome: Pain in

162

the face, aggravated by physical strain, flushing of face, dizziness, tinnitus, poor appetite, irritability, dry stools, red tongue with little coating, and a fine and rapid pulse.

(2) Therapeutic methods:

① Obstruction of Wind and Cold syndrome:

Prescription: Zanzhu (BL 2), Sibai (ST 2), Xiaguan (ST 7), Waiguan (SJ 5), and Hegu (LI 4).

Manipulation: Puncture by adopting filiform needles with reducing method.

② Excess Heat in Yangming channel syndrome:

Prescription: Taiyang (EX-HN5), Sibai (ST 2), Xiaguan (ST 7), Neiting (ST 44), and Zusanli (ST 36).

Manipulation: Puncture by using filiform needles with reducing method.

③ Hyperactivity of Yang due to Yin Deficiency syndrome:

Prescription: Zanzhu (BL 2), Sibai (ST 2), Xiaguan (ST 7), Fengchi (GB 20), Taixi (KI 3), and Taichong LR 3).

Manipulation: Puncture by using filiform needles with reducing method except for Taixi (KI 3) which is treated with reinforcing method.

(3) Other therapy:

Auricular acupuncture: Select Forehead (EP-E9), Upper Jaw (EP-A7), Shenmen (EP-I1) and Sympathetic (EP-H1) to be needled with strong stimulation, 2-3 points each time. The needles should be retained for 20-30 minutes during which they are manipulated once every 5 minutes. Needling-embedding is applicable.

2. Facial neuritis

This is an acute, non-pyogenic inflammation of the facial nerves in the stylomastoid foramen, which often causes peripheral facial paralysis. Its exact causes are unknown. This disease may occur in the population of any age, but mostly in those between 20-40 years old, and its incidence is a little higher in females than in males. In most cases, it is bilateral and usually has an acute onset marked by sudden paralysis of the mimetic muscle of one side, which may reach its peak within several hours. In TCM, it is called "deviation of the mouth and eyes" or simply "deviation of mouth".

(1) Syndrome identification:

Affection of exogenous pathogenic Wind syndrome: Sudden deviation of the mouth and eyes, which is mostly found in the morning when the patient is to dress up with numbness in one side of the face or pain in the retroauricular region, swelling and pain in the inferoauricular region or in the face and deviation of the mouth corner toward the healthy side as its early symptoms. These symptoms are then accompanied with disappearance of the wrinkles on the forehead, shallowness of the labionasal grooves, stuffy nose, failure to shut eyes, lacrimination, inability of the mouth to be tightly shut while blowing, red tongue with thin and whitish coating, and a floating, rapid or floating and tense pulse.

② Stirring of endogenous Wind of Deficiency type: Sudden deviation of the mouth and eyes, flushing of face, dizziness, tinnitus, or decline or disappearance of the tasting sense in the anterior part of the tongue, stiffiness of the tongue root, deviation of the tongue toward the healthy side, dark red tongue with a whitish coating, and a wiry pulse.

(2) Therapeutic method:

Affection of exogenous pathogenic Wind syndrome:

Prescription: Fengchi (GB 20), Dicang (ST 4), Jiache (ST 6), Sibai (ST 2), Yangbai (BL 14), Hegu (LI 4), and Yifeng (SJ 18).

Manipulation: Puncture by adopting filiform needles with reducing method on Fengchi (GB 20), reinforcing method and then the reducing method on Zusanli (ST 36), Taichong (LR 3), Sanyinjiao (SP 6). The rest points are treated with reinforcing method penetrately in combination with moxibustion with moxa roll.

(3) Other therapies:

① Auricular acupuncture: Select Cheeks (EP-A11), Liver (EP-N9), Eyes (EP-A10), Mouth (EP-M1), Subcortex (EP-E10) and Adrenal Gland (EP-B8) to be needled with strong stimulation, 3-5 points each time with the needles retained for 30-60 minutes, once every other day. Needle-embedding is applicable.

② Electric acupuncture: Select Dicang (ST 4), Jiache (ST 6),

Yangbai (BG 14) and Hegu (LI 4) to be needled with the electric acupuncture instrument with an intensity of low frequency that arouses a comfort feeling or mild vibration of the facial muscles in patient. The needles are retained for 5-10 minutes. This therapy is suitable for patients with a longer history and contraindicated for the disease at the acute stage.

3. Intercostal neuralgia

Intercostal neuralgia refers to the recurrent pain in the area where one or several intercostal nerves are distributed, which is episodically aggravated or induced or aggravated by deep inhalation, cough or sneezing. It often results from herpes zoster or from diseases of the adjacent organs and tissues. In TCM, it is called "hypochondriac pain".

(1) Syndrome identification:

① Stagnation of the Liver Qi syndrome: Migratory pain in the costal region which is often induced or aggravated by emotional upset, chest fullness, eructation,, thin and whitish tongue coating and a wiry and forceful pulse.

② Blood Stasis syndrome: Fixed prickle-like pain in the costal region, a history of chronic pain in the costal region or taumatic injury, distending pain with ternderness or palpable mass in the hypochondriac region, purplish dark tongue which may be dotted with ecchymosis, and a deep uneven pulse.

③ Yin Deficiency syndrome: Migratory dull pain in the costal region, aggravated by changing body position or physical strain, lustreless face, red cheeks, lower fever, dizziness, vertigo, reddened tongue with little coating, and a fine and rapid pulse.

(2) Therapeutic methods:

① Stagnation of the Liver Qi syndrome:

Prescription: Zhongting (RN 16), Ganshu (BL 18), Qimen (LR 14), Xiaxi (GB 43).

Manipulation: Puncture by using filiform needles with reducing method.

② Blood Stasis syndrome:

Prescription: Dabao (SP 21), Jingmen (GB 25), Xingjian (LR

2), Geshu (BL 17), Sanyinjiao (SP 6).

Manipulation: Puncture by using filiform needles with reducing method.

③ Yin Deficiency syndrome:

Prescription: Yinxi (HT 6), Xinshu (BL 15), Xuehai (SP 10), Sanyinjiao (SP 6).

Manipulation: Puncture by using filiform needles with reinforcing method.

4. Sciatica

This is a group of painful symptoms appearing in the distribution route of the sciatic nerve, or the lumbar region, the gluteal region, the posterior aspects of the thign and leg and the lateral side of the foot. It is classified as two types: The primary and the secondary. The primary sciatica, also known as sciatic neuritis, is a sciatica with unknown reasons; while the secondary sciatica is usually caused by compress or stimuli of the adjacent tissues in the distribution route of the nerve, especially that of the protrusion of the lumbar intervertebral disc, lumbar or sacral meningitis and sacro-iliilis. This disease usually affects the young and the middle aged males and in most cases, it is bilateral. Clinically it may attack suddenly or slowly and is manifested as aching in the lower back or the premonitory symptoms of the disease such as a feeling of stiffiness in the back or the lower back in the case of its acute onset. The typical sciatica presents a pain that radiates to the distal end from the gluteal region to the posterior aspect of the thign, the lateral sides of the popliteal fossa and the leg in sequence, being burning or scorching or cutting pain in nature. In TCM, it is known as "arthralgia syndrome" or "pain in the loins and knees".

(1) Syndrome identification:

① Obstruction of Cold-Dampness in the collaterals syndrome: Pain with a cold and a heavy sensation or as being prickleded or splitted in severe cases in the loins and leg, aggravated by exposure to cold and not relieved by lying flat, difficulty in moving the affected leg, pale tongue with a white and greasy tongue coating, and a deep, tense or deep slow pulse.

② Obstruction of Dampness-Heat in the collaterals syndrome:
Soreness, numbness and distending pain in the lower back and the
leg, or even a burning or scorching sensation in severe cases, difficulty of the affected leg in movement, vexation, thirst, red tongue
with yellow coating, and a wiry rapid pulse.

③ Blockage by Blood Stasis in the interior syndrome: Lumbago
with the painful area being aggravated by pressing initially, followed
by radiating pain that involves the posterior aspect of the thign or
the heel. The pain is usually aggravated by cough, defecation or
walk, and relieved by flexing the knees in a sitting or a lying position. The tongue is usually purplish and dark in colour or dotted
with ecchymosis, and the pulse is deep and uneven.

(2) Therapeutic methods:

① Obstruction of Cold-Dampness in the collaterals syndrome:

Prescription: Shenshu (BL 23), Dachangshu (BL 25), Zhibian
(BL 54), Huantiao (GB 30), Yinmen (BL 37), Weizhong (BL 40),
Kunlun (BL 60), and Yanglingquan (GB 34).

Manipulation: Puncture by adopting filiform needle with reducing
method. Moxibustion is applied to Shenshu (BL 23) additionally.

② Obstruction of Dampness-Heat in the collaterals syndrome:

Prescription: Pangguangshu (BL 28), Zhibian (BL 54), Huantiao (GB 30), Fengshi (GB 31), Weizhong (BL 40), Yanglingquan
(GB 34), Feiyang (BL 58), and Kunlun (BL 60).

Manipulation: Puncture by using filiform needles with reducing
method.

③ Blockage by Blood Stasis in the interior syndrome:

Prescription: Jiaji (EX-B2) at the level of the painful area, Zhibian (BL 54), Ciliao (BL 32), Huantiao (GB 30), Yinmen (BL 37),
Weizhong (BL 40), Kunlun (BL 60).

Manipulation: Puncture by using filiform needles with reinforcing
method and then the reducing method.

(3) Other therapies:

① Auricular acupuncture: Select Sciatic Nerve (EP-H2), Hip
(EP-H3), Shenmen (EP-I1), Adrenal Gland (EP-B8) and Lumbar
Vertebra (EP-F3) to be needled with moderate or strong stimula-

tion. The needles are retained for 10-30 minutes during which the needles are manipulated once every 5 minutes. The treatment is done once every day or every other day. The points may also be treated by needle-embedding.

② Electric acupuncture: Select Shenshu (BL 23), Dachangshu (BL 25), Weizhong (BL 40), Zhibian (BL 54), Chengshan (BL 57), Kunlun (BL 60), Huantiao (GB 30), Fengshi (GB 31) and Yanglingquan (GB 34) to be needled, 2-3 points are used each time with a stimulation of high frequency and continuous waves that patient can bear, once daily or once every other day. The needles are retained for 20-30 minutes.

5. Cerebrovascular diseases

Cerebrovascular disease is a collective term for the cerebral lesions arising from vascular diseases. It is marked by disturbance of the local cerebral blood circulation or function of cerebral region that develops rapidly from various kinds of disorders of the cerebral vessels, especially the rupture or obstruction of the arteries, which often gives rise to cerebral bleeding, subarachnoid cavity or cerebral embolism. This disease usually occurs in patients after the middle age who usually have a history of hypertension or atherosclerosis. Clinically, it has a sudden onset and rapid progression, with coma, hemiplegia and aphasia as its main symptoms. After the acute stage, severe sequela often follows. The disease can be divided into two types: The hamorralgic and the ischemic, and, in TCM, it is called "affection of Wind".

(1) Syndrome identification:

① Affection of the channel and collateral:

Invasion of Wind pathogen into the empty collaterals: Numbness of the skin, muscles and the limbs, sudden occurrence of deviation of the eyes and mouth, cluttering, salivation with drops from the corner of mouth or hemiplegia, thin and whitish tongue coating, and a floating and rapid pulse.

Up-stirring of hyperactive Liver Yang due to Deficiency of both the Liver-Yin and the Kidney-Yin syndrome: Original headache, dizziness, tinnitus, vertigo, insomnia with dream-disturbed sleep,

168

soreness and weakness of the loins and knees, sudden occurrence of numbness and heaviness of unilateral limbs, deviation of eyes and mouth, hemiplegia, stiffness of tongue with aphasia, red tongue with thin yellow or white greasy coating, and a wiry slippery or a wiry, fine and rapid pulse.

② Affection of the Zang-Fu organs:

The Bi syndrome of apoplexy: Sudden coma, lockjaw, clenched fist, red face, coarse breathing, rales in the throat, constipation, oliguria, yellow greasy tongue coating, and a wiry, slippery and rapid or a forceful wiry pulse.

The Tuo syndrome of apoplexy: Sudden coma with the mouth opened and the eyes shut, snoring, feeble breath, entension of the fingers, cold limbs, incontinence of urine and stools, profuse oily sweat, hemiplegia, deviation of the tongue, feeble and indistinct pulse.

③ Sequela: If the disease is not fully cured in six months, it will remain such sequelas as hemiplegia or cluttering.

Hemiplegia: This is mostly caused by Deficiency of Qi and obstruction of the collaterals due to Blood Stasis, which is marked by weakness, flaccidity and dysfunction, or convulsion and difficulty in movement of the affected limbs.

Muttering: This is usually ascribed to Wind-Phlegm in the collaterals, which is manifested as deviation of the tongue, stiffness of the tongue root, muttering, forgetfulness, liability to laugh, white greasy tongue coating, and a wiry greasy or a soft greasy pulse.

(2) Therapeutic methods:

① Affection of the channel and collateral:

Invasion of Wind pathogen into the empty collaterals:

Prescription: Zusanli (ST 36), Sanyinjiao (SP 6), Baihui (DU 20), Fengchi (GB 20), Waiguan (SJ 5), Hegu (LI 4), Taichong (LR 3), Yanglingquan (GB 34), Huantiao (GB 30), Fengshi (GB 31), Yangbai (GB 14), Sibai (ST 2), Yingxiang (LI 20), Jiache (ST 36), and Dicang (ST 4).

Manipulation: Puncture by adopting filiform needles with reinforcing method on Zusanli (ST 36), Sanyinjiao (SP 6) and Baihui

(DU 20), with reducing method on Fengchi (GB 20) and Taichong (LR 3), and with the uniform reinforcing and reducing method on the rest points.

Up-stirring of hyperactive Liver Yang due to Deficiency of both the Liver-Yin and the Kidney yin:

Prescription: Taichong (LR 3), Sanyinjiao (SP 6), Shuigou (DU 26), Laogong (PC 8), Zusanli (ST 36). For cases with paralysis in the upper limb, add Waiguan (SJ 5), Hegu (LI 4), Jianyu (LI 15) and Jianliao (SJ 14); for cases with paralysis in the lower limbs, add Fengshi (GB 31), Yanglingquan (GB 34) and Kunlun (BL 60); and for cases with deviation of eyes and mouth, add Dicang(ST 4), Jiache (ST 6), Yangbai (GB 14), Zanzhu (BL 2) and Yanglao (SI 6).

Manipulation: Puncture by adopting filiform needles with reducing method on Taichong (LR 3), Shuigou (DU 26), Waiguan (SJ 5), Hegu (LI 4), reinforcing method on Taixi (KI 3), Zusanli (ST 36) and Sanyinjiao (SP 6), and the uniform reinforcing and reducing method on the rest points.

② Affection of Zang-Fu organs:

The Bi syndrome of apoplexy:

Prescription: Shuigou (DU 26), Taichong (LR 3), Fenglong (ST 40), Laogong (PC 8), and the twelve Jing-Well points.

Manipulation: Puncture by using filiform needles with reducing method or prick to cause bleeding.

The Tuo syndrome of apoplexy:

Prescription: Guanyuan (RN 4) and Shenque (RN 8).

Manipulation: Moxibustion with large moxa cones.

③ Sequela:

Hemiplegia:

Prescription: Zusanli (ST 36), Shenshu (BL 23), Sanyinjiao (SP 6), Xuehai (SP 10), Guanyuan (RN 4). Add Jianyu (LI 15), Hegu (LI 4), Quchi (LI 11) and Waiguan (SJ 5) for cases with paralysis in the upper limb, Huantiao (GB 30), Yanglingquan (GB 34), Jiexi (ST 41), Kunlun (BL 60) for cases with paralysis in the lower limbs, Yangbai (GB 14), Dicang (ST 4), Jiache (ST 6), Yingxiang

(LI 20) and Chengjiang (RN 24) for cases with deviation of eyes and mouth.

Manipulation: Puncture by adopting filiform needles with reinforcing method on Zusanli (ST 36), Shenshu (BL 23), Sanyinjiao (SP 6), Xuehai (SP 10), Guanyuan (RN 4), Yanglingquan (GB 34), and Jiexi (ST 41), and the uniform reinforcing and reducing method on the rest points.

Mutterring:

Prescription: Fenglong (ST 40), Zusanli (ST 36), Shenmen (HT 7), Neiguan (PC 6), Lianquan (RN 23), Tongli (HT 5), Yamen (DU 15), Tiantu (RN 22) and Zhaohai (KI 6).

Manipulation: Puncture by using filiform needles with reducing method on Fenglong (ST 40), Neiguan (PC 6) and Tongli (HT 5), and the uniform reinforcing and reducing method on the rest points.

(3) Other therapies:

① Scalp acupuncture: Select Anterior Oblique Line of Vertex Temporal (MS 6), Posterior Oblique Line of vertex temporal (MS 7), Lateral Line 1 of vertex (MS 8), Lateral Line 2 of vertex (MS 9), Anterior Temporal Line (MS 10) and Posterior Temporal Line (MS 11) to be needled 0. 5-1 cun subcutaneously with the needles retained for 20-30 minutes, once every day.

② Electric acupuncture: Select Jianyu (LI 15), Quchi (LI 11), Waiguan (SJ 5), Hegu (LI 4), Huantiao (GB 30), Fengshi (GB 31), Yanglingquan (GB 34), Xuanzhong (GB 39) for cases with sequela of hemiplegia, one pair of points on the upper and the lower limbs respectively each time, to be needled with the electric acupuncture instrument by exerting sparse-intense waves of low frequency. The needles are remained 20-30 minutes, and the treatment is done once a day.

6. Hysteria

Hysteria is one of the commonly seen neuroses, which is often seen in young females. It is a paroxysmal and recurrent disease marked by hypertension of the advance nervous system and temporary dysfunction of the cerebrum by reasons of emotional factors. Its clinical manifestations are complicated and variable. It is often manifested as disturbance of the spirit, motor and sense, or dysfunction of the vegetative nerves or the visceral organs, but no positive founding can be revealed by examinations. Usually it has a sudden onset and disappears quickly, and suggestion often induces and changes the disease's conditions or leads to its disappearance. Some patients are liable for emotional changes originally, tending to exaggerate things, affected or hinted and illusive, and like to show himself off. In TCM, this disease is called "restlessness of Zang organ", "mental depression" or "lily disease".

(1) Syndrome identification:

① Stagnation of Qi syndrome: Mental depression, eructation, disinclination to talk, sitting long with an disinterested complexion, lethargy, liability to lie flat, obstructing feeling in the throat, pale tongue with white or greasy coating, and a deep, wiry pulse.

② Wind-Phlegm syndrome: Sudden coma, or sleeping with semiunconsciousness, rales in the throat, vomiting foamy vomitus, rigidity of the limbs, red tongue with whitish coating and a wiry and slippery pulse.

③ Restlessness of visceral organ syndrome: Laughing and crying alternately, beating his/her chest and stamping his/her feet, or trance, hyperactivity of the limbs, rigidity of the limbs which fail to move voluntarily or even convulsion or paralysis, false blindness, aphasia or deafness, pale tongue with whitish and greasy coating, and a wiry, slippery and rapid or a tense pulse.

(2) Therapeutic methods:

① Stagnation of Qi syndrome:

Prescription: Taichong (LR 3), Xingjian (LR 2), Shenmen (HT 7), Daling (PC 7), Sanyinjiao (SP 6) and Yongquan (KI 1).

Manipulation: Puncture by using filiform needles with reducing method on Taichong (LR 3), Xingjian (LR 2) and Daling (PC 7), and the uniform reinforcing and reducing method on the rest points.

② Wind-Phlegm syndrome:

Prescription: Renzhong (RN 26), Neiguan (PC 6), Fenglong (ST 40), Zhongwan (RN 12), Taichong (LR 4), and Yanglingquan (GB 34).

Manipulation: Puncture by adopting filiform needles with reducing method.

③ Restlessness of visceral organ syndrome:

Prescription: Renzhong (RN 26), Neiguan (PC 6), Baihui (DU 20), Shenmen (HT 7), Yongquan (KI 1), and Taichong (LR 3).

Manipulation: Puncture by using filiform needles with reducing method.

(3) Other therapy:

Auricular acupuncture: Select Liver (EP-N9), Heart (EP-O1), Shenmen (EP-I1), Subcortex (EP-E10), Sympathetic (EP-H1) and Occiput (EP-E5) to be needled with strong stimulation. After the needles are constantly twisted for 5 minutes, remain the needles for 30-40 minutes until the symptoms disappear and the patients get calm.

Surgical Diseases

1. Abdominal fluctuance after operation

This is a disease caused by temporal paralysis of the intestine due to stimuli of an operation, which is mainly manifested as abdominal fullness, inability to eat, nausea, absence of defecation or windbreak, and diminution or disappearance of the bowel sound. It usually appears 2-5 days after operation.

(1) Therapeutic method:

Prescription: Zusanli (ST 36), Zhongwan (RN 12), Tianshu (ST 25), Shenque (RN 8).

Manipulation: Puncture by using filiform needles with a weak reinforcing method except for Shenque (RN 8) which is treated by warming moxibustion.

(2) Other therapy:

Auricular acupuncture: Select Large intestine (EP-M8), Small intestine (EP-M 6), Stomach (EP-M4), Spleen (EP-N10) and Sympathetic (EP-H1) to be needled with strong stimulation. The needles are remained for 1-2 hours.

2. Acute mastitis

Acute mastitis is an acute pyogenic diseases of the breast which often occurs following rupture of the nipple, or infection of staphylococcus or streptococcus during lactation. It is mostly seen in the primipara and usually occurs 2-5 weeks after delivery. At the initial stage, it is manifested as chills, fever, swelling and pain of the affected breast with redness, hard nodule and obvious tenderness in a local area of the breast. In TCM, it is called "breast abscess" or "blowing of breast".

(1) Syndrome identification:

Accumulation of Dampness-Heat syndrome: Pain, swelling and nodule of the affected breast, unsmooth discharge of milk, chills, fever, thirst, poor apetite, yellow and greasy tongue coating, and a slippery rapid or a floating rapid pulse.

(2) Therapeutic method:

Accumulation of Dampness-Heat syndrome:

Prescription: Jianjing (GB 21), Shaoze (SI 1), Shanzhong (RN 17), Rugen (ST 18), Zusanli (ST 36), Neiguan (PC 6) and Quchi (LI 11).

Manipulation: Puncture with reducing method by filiform needles. For cases with high fever, add Dazhui (DU 14) and Hegu (LI 4) to be needled.

(3) Other therapy:

Moxibustion: Cut a Chinese garlic into slices or pound the garlic into paste to be applied to the affected area, then apply the warming moxibustion for 10-20 minutes, once or twice a day.

3. Periarthritis of the shoulder

Periarthritis of the shoulder is a degenerative and inflammatory diseases of the capsule of the shoulder joint and its surrounding soft tissues, mostly seen in the females from 40 to 60 years old. This disease is mainly marked by irradiative, diffusive and stationary pain of the shoulder, with pain as its main symptom at its early stage and dysfunction of the shoulder joint at the later stage. In TCM, it is called " Exposure of the shoulder to Wind" or " stagnancy in shoulder. "

① Wind-Cold syndrome: Sudden onset, fixed and severe pain, which is aggravated by exposure to cold and relieved by warmth, difficulty of the shoulder joint in movements, normal skin colour without a hot feeling on palpation in the affected area, thin and whitish tongue coating, and a wiry tense pulse.

② Wind-Dampness syndrome: Soreness, heaviness, fixed pain and mild swelling in the affected area, numbness of the skin and muscles in the shoulder region, difficulty of the shoulder joint in movement, heavy sensation of the both hands, white and greasy tongue coating and a soft and moderate pulse.

③ Loss of nourishment of the tendons syndrome: Protractable shoulder pain, failure to lift the arm above the head or to touch the back, soreness and pain in the shoulder, lassitude, aversion to cold which can be relieved by warmth and aggravated by cold in the affected area, pale tongue with thin and whitish coating, and a fine pulse.

(2) Therapeutic methods:

① Wind-Cold syndrome:

Prescription: Jianyu (LI 15), Jianliao (SJ 14), Jianzhen (SI 9), Hegu (LI 4).

Manipulation: Puncture by using filiform needles with the reducing method on Hegu (LI 4) and the uniform reinforcing and reducing method on the rest points which are also treated by warm moxibustion.

② Wind-Dampness syndrome:

Prescription: Jianyu (LI 15), Jugu (LI 16), Quchi (LI 11), Zusanli (ST 36), and Tianzong (SI 11).

Manipulation: Puncture by using filiform needles with reducing method on Quchi (LI 11), the reinforcing method on Zusanli (ST 36), and the uniform reinforcing and reducing method on the rest points which are also treated by moxibustion with moxa roll.

③ Loss of nourishment of the tendons syndrome:

Prescription: Jianyu (LI 15), Jianliao (SJ 14), Jianzhen (SI 9), Dazhu (BL 11), Tianzong (SI 11), Quchi (LI 11), Yanglingquan

(GB 34).

Manipulation: Puncture by adopting filiform needles with reinforcing method. The local points are treated with strong stimulation
in combination with warming moxibustion.

(3) Other therapies:

① Scalp acupuncture: Posterior oblique line of vertex-temporal
(MS 7) of the opposite side, Lateral line 1 of vertex (MS 8) and the
Lateral line 2 of vertex (MS 9) of the opposite side, to be needled
subcutaneously 1-1. 5 cun, with the needles retained for 20-30 minutes, once daily.

② Electric acupuncture: Select Jianyu (LI 15), Jianliao (SJ 14),
Jianzhen (SI 9), and Quchi (LI 11) to be needled with electric
acupuncture instrument by applying continuous waves of high frequency. The needles are retained for 20-30 minutes, and the treatment is resumed once daily.

4. External humeral epicondylitis

This refers to non-bacterial inflammation of the external humeral
epicondyle, the head of humerus, and the humeroradial joint, also
known popularly as tennis elbow. It is mostly caused by injury to
the starting part of the radial flexor muscle due to improper exertion
of force while the forearm is rotating. The disease is marked by pain
around the external humeral epicondyle and the humeroradial joints
which is aggravated when the forearm is in a rotating position or a
fist is made hardly. In TCM, it is called "elbow strain", or "obstruction of vessels in the bone".

(1) Therapeutic method:

Prescription: Zhouliao (LI 12) and Hegu (LI 4).

Manipulation: Puncture by adopting filiform needles with reducing method.

(2) Other therapy:

Moxibustion: Select Ah Shi points to be treated with warm moxibustion for 10-20 minutes, or with moxibustion with ginger for 3-7
Zhuang, once or twice a day.

5. Stiff neck

Stiff neck is an acute simple disease marked by rigidity and pain with limited movement in the neck, seen mostly in adults. It is mostly caused by long-standing over extension of the muscles of the neck which further results in spasm of the muscles, or by incarceration of the synovium or semi-dislocation of the minor cervical articulations, or inflammation of the muslces and tendons. Clinically it is manifested as failure to turn the head or look upward, sudden occurrence of soreness, pain and rigidity of the muscles of the neck, which is accompanied with notable ternderness and can be relieved by hot compress. In TCM, it is called "disease caused by improper height of pillow" or "injury to tendon of the neck".

(1) Therapeutic method:

Prescription: Luozhenxue (located on the ulnar border of the second metacarpophalangeal joints when a fist is made slightly), Fengchi (GB 20), Houxi (SI 3) and Xuanzhong (GB 39).

Manipulation: Puncture by using filiform needles with reducing method. Moxibustion is adopted in combination for the local points.

(2) Other therapies:

① Moxibustion: Select Dazhui (DU 14), Tianzhu (BL 10), Fengchi (GB 20) and the Ah Shi points to be treated by moxibustion with moxa roll until the skin gets flush.

② Auricular acupuncture: Select Neck (EP-F5), Cervical vertebrae (EP-F1), Shenmen (EP-I1), Subcortex (EP-E10) and Liver (EP-N9), 2-3 points each time, to be treated by twisting the needles rapidly after they are inserted. The needles are retained for 20-30 minutes during which they are manipulated once every 5 or 10 minutes. Resume the treatment once daily.

6. Cervical spondylopathy

This refers to a group of symptoms produced by pathological changes of the cervical vertebrae and their surrounding soft tissues including the intervertebral discs, the yellow ligament and the synovium of the spinal cord, which stimulate or press the roots of the cervical nerves, the spinal cord, the vertebral artery and the sympathetic nerve. It mostly affects the males of the middle aged or the aged, with pain in the neck, shoulder and arm, numbness of the upper limbs, limitation of the movement of the neck, or accompanied with dizziness, nausea, vomiting, tinnitus, deafness or blurred vision, or even disturbance of movements or spasmodic paralysis in the upper and the lower limbs as its main clinical manifestations. It can be divided into the cervical type, type of the root of the cervical nerves, type of the cervical spinal cord, type of the cerbical sympathetic nerve, and the vertebral artery type. In TCM, it is called "arthralgia syndrome'.

(1) Syndrome identification:

① Wind-Cold syndrome: Rigidity of the neck and headache, inability to turn the head freely, aversion to cold, no sweating or sweating, aching in the shoulder, back or the four limbs, which is more severe in the upper limbs, thin whitish tongue coating, and a floating moderate or a floating and tense pulse.

② Affection of Wind, Cold and Dampness syndrome: Fixed pain in the head, the neck, the shoulder, the back and the limbs, which is relieved by warmth and aggravated by cold, stiff neck with limited movement, streak-like nodules palpated in the posterior aspect of the neck, heaviness, numbness and weakness in the upper limbs which may be complicated by atrophy of muscles, enlarged tongue with teethmarks, deep slow or wiry and slippery pulse.

③ Stagnation of Qi and Blood Stasis syndrome: Stabbling and fixed pain with ternderness in the head, the neck, the shoulder, the back and the limbs, muscular atrophy of hands, numbness of the tips of the fingers with a blue-purplish skin colour, depression of nails without lustre, dry and itching skin, or even convulsion or spasm of the muscles of the limbs, or dizziness, vertigo, rough and dequamous skin, lustreless face, purplish and dark tongue which may be dotted with ecchymosis, and a fine, uneven or a wiry and uneven pulse.

④ Interlocking of Phlegm and Blood Stasis syndrome: Dizziness, vertigo, heavy sensation over head as if being bound, a feeling of obstruction of foreign body in the throat, weak and heavy limbs, enlarged, dark and purplish tongue or dotted with ecchymosis, white greasy tongue coating, and a wiry pulse, in addition to the symptoms of stagnation of Qi and Blood Stasis.

⑤ Deficiency of both the Liver and the Kidney syndrome: Dizziness, vertigo, tinnitus, deafness, flushing of face, feverish sensation over the palms, soles and chest, insomnia, dream-disturbed sleep, irritability, soreness and weakness of the loins and knees, muscular twitching and cramp, red tongue with little coating, and a fine and rapid pulse.

(2) Therapeutic methods:

① Wind-Cold syndrome:

Prescription: Dazhui (DU 14), Tianzhu (BL 10), Jianwaishu (SI 14), Xuanzhong (BL 39) and Houxi (SI 3).

Manipulation: Puncture by using filiform needles with reducing method in the case that the syndrome is an exterior excessive one, and with uniform reinforcing and reducing method in the case that the syndrome is an exterior Deficiency one.

② Affection of Wind, Cold and Dampness syndrome:

Prescription: Dazhui (DU 14), Fengchi (GB 20), Tianzhu (BL 10), Jianjing (GB 21), Waiguan (SJ 5), and the Jiaji points (EX-B2) corresponding to the diseased location.

Manipulation: Puncture by using filiform needles with strong reducing method or uniform reinforcing and reducing method in patients with a weak constitution.

③ Stagnation of Qi and Blood Stasis syndrome:

Prescription: Cervical Jiaji points (EX-B2) corresponding to the disease location, Bailao (EX-HN 15), Dazhui (DU 14), Jianjing (GB 21), Jianyu (LI 15), Yanglao (SI 6), Tiaokou (ST 38), and Geshu (BL 17).

Manipulation: Puncture by adopting filiform needles with reducing method of moderate stimulation or uniform reinforcing and reducing method except for Yanglao (SI 6) which should be treated with strong reducing method.

④ Interlocking of Phlegm and Blood Stasis syndrome:

Prescription: Cervical Jiaji points (EX-B 2) corresponding to the disease location, Dazhui (DU 14), Jianjing (GB 21), Jianyu (LI 15), Zusanli (ST 36), Geshu (BL 17), and Fenglong (ST 40).

Manipulation: Puncture by using filiform needles with reducing method. But in patients with general weakness, the uniform reinforcing and reducing method or the reinforcing method should be adopted.

⑤ Deficiency of both the Liver and the Kidney syndrome:

Prescription: Dazhui (DU 14), Lingtai (DU 10), Ganshu (BL 18), Shenshu (BL 23), Yanglingquan (GB 34), Xuanzhong (GB 39), Yanglao (SI 6).

Manipulation: Puncture mainly with uniform reinforcing and reducing method. In the case of spasm of the limbs, the points on the limbs should be needled with reducing method.

(3) Other therapies:

① Electric acupuncture: Select Bailao (EX-HN 150), Dazhui (DU 14), Fengchi (GB 20), Dazhu (BL 1), Jianjing (GB 21) and Jugu (LI 16), 2-4 points each time, to be needled with the electric acupuncture instrument by using countinuous waves of high frequency, once daily. The needles are retained for 20 minutes.

② Auricular acupuncture: Select Neck (EP-F5), Cervical vertebra (EP-F1), Shoulder (EP-J4), Sympathetic (EP-H1), Adrenal gland (EP-B8), Liver (EP-N9), Kidney (EP-N4), 2-3 points each time, to be treated with strong stimulation with the needle retained for 20 minutes, once daily or once every other day.

7. Acute sprain of the lumbar muscle

The acute sprain of the lumbar muscle is a disease with lumbago and limited movement of the loins as its main symptoms which are caused by sudden injury to the soft tissues of the lumbar region. It mostly occurs in the case of an improper posture being taken while bearing heavy loading, improper exertion of force or fall and contusion. In TCM, it is called "lumbago" or "injury to tendon".

(1) Therapeutic method:

Prescription: Shuigou (DU 26), Shenshu (B 23), Weizhong (BL 40), and Houxi (SI 3).

Manipulation: Puncture with filiform needles with reducing method. Weizhong (BL 40) may also be treated by pricking to cause bleeding.

(2) Other therapy:

180

Auricular acupuncture: Select Lumbar vertebra (EP-F3), Shenmen (EP-I1), Adrenal gland (EP-B8) and Subcortex (EP-E10) to be needled with strong stimulation, once daily or once every other day with the needle retained for 30-60 minutes.

Gynecological and Pediatric Diseases

1. Dysmenorrhea

Dysmenorrhea is a symptom marked by spasmodic abdominal pain around menstruation, which can be divided into either the primary or the secondary. The former refers to the dysmenorrhea that has occurred at the first menstruation of one's life, which is often caused by maldevelopment of the uterus or disorders of the endocrine system; while the latter indicates the dysmenorrhea that occurs 2 years later after the first menstruation, which is mostly related to diseases of the internal genitalia in the pelvic cavity. Clinically, it is manifested as colicky, stabbling or distending pain in the lower abdomen, often accompanied with soreness and weakness of the loins and knees, headache, vomiting, etc. It is a common young female disease, and in TCM it is called "dysmenorrhea" or "abdominal pain during menstruation."

(1) Syndrome identification:

① Stagnation of Cold-Dampness syndrome: Cold pain in the lower abdomen before or during menstruation, aggravated by pressure or referring to the lower back, or relieved by warmth, scanty dark menses which is often mixed with blood clots, thin and whitish tongue coating and a deep tense pulse.

② Stagnation of Qi and Blood Stasis syndrome: More distension and pain in the lower abdomen before or during menstruation, little mense, dribbling of the menses which is dark purplish in colour, mixed with blood clots or takes an appearance of rotten meat, alleviation of pain after menstruation, accompanied with distending pain in the chest, costal region, and the breats, dark purplish tongue which may be dotted with ecchymosis, thin tongue coating and a deep wiry pulse.

③ Deficiency of both Qi and Blood syndrome: Dull pain in the lower abdomen during or after menstruation, which is relieved by pressure, thin and light coloured mense, pale complexion, listlessness, pale tongue with thin coating, and a feeble and fine pulse.

④ Depletion of the Liver and the Kidney syndrome: Dull pain in the lower abdomen during or after menstruation, scanty mense which is light in colour, sorness and pain in the back and the lower back, dizziness, tinnitus, reddish tougue with a thin coating, and a deep, fine pulse.

(2) Therapeutic methods:

① Stagnation of Cold-Dampness syndrome:

Prescription: Zhongji (RN 3), Shuidao (ST 28), and Diji (SP 8).

Manipulation: Puncture by using filiform needles with reducing method, then apply moxibustion with moxa roll on these points.

② Stagnation of Qi and Blood Stasis syndrome:

Prescription: Qihai (RN 6), Taichong (LR 3), Sanyinjiao (SP 6), and Xuehai (SP 10).

Manipulation: Puncture by using filiform needles with reducing method.

③ Deficiency of both Qi and Blood syndrome:

Prescription: Pishu (BL 20), Weishu (BL 21), Zusanli (ST 36).

Manipulation: Puncture by using filiform needles with reinforcing method, then apply moxibustion with moxa cone for a period of 5-7 cones being burnt.

④ Depletion of the Liver and the Kidney syndrome:

Prescription: Ganshu (BL 18), Shenshu (BL 23), and Guanyuan (RN 4).

Manipulation: Puncture by using filiform needles and apply warming moxibustion with moxa roll after the puncturing.

(3) Other thearpy:

Auricular therapy: Select Uterus (EP-I 5), Endocrine (EP-O1), Sympathetic (EP-H1), Shenmen (EP-I1), Subcortex (EP-E10) and

182

Kidney (EP-N4), 2-4 points each time, to be needled with moderate or strong stimulation, once daily. The needles are retained for 20 minutes.

2. Dysfunctional uterine bleeding

This refers to abnormal bleeding of the endometrium due to disorder of the endocrine system which presents no organic lesions on gynecological examinations. It has two types: The anovulatory dysfunctional uterine bleeding and the ovulatory uterine bleeding. The former is caused by dysfunction of the ovulation and is usually seen in women of adolescence or climacteric; while the latter is caused by dysfunction of the yellow body of ovary which usually affects the women of child-bearing age. Clinically, it is mainly manifested as irregular menstrual period, menorrahgia, menostaxis, dribbling of blood, etc., which mostly arise from disturbance of any link of the central nervous system and the hypothalamus-pituitary-ovary axis. In TCM, it is called "metrostaxis and metrorrhagia".

(1) Syndrome identification:

① Excessive Heat syndrome: Menorrhagia which is purplish or dark red in colour, fetid in ordour, thick and mixed with blood clots, abdominal pain with ternderness, constipation, thirst, red tongue with yellow coating and a wiry, rapid and forceful pulse.

② Yin Deficiency syndrome: Bright red blood, dizziness, tinnitus, palpitation, insomnia, tidal fever in the afternoon, red tongue without coating, and fine, rapid and forceless pulse.

③ Qi Deficiency syndrome: Prolonged disease course, light coloured or dark extravasated blood, pain with a cold feeling in the lower abdomen, pale and puffy face, listlessness and lassitude, lethargy, poor appetite, white tongue coating with much fluid, and a fine and slow pulse.

④ Collapse syndrome: Metrorrhagia, followed by faint, pale face, profuse cold perspiration, rapid breathing, cold limbs, and a feeble and indistinct pulse.

(2) Therapeutic method:

Prescription: Guanyuan (RN 4), Sanyinjiao (SP 6), Yinbai (SP 1). For cases with excessive Heat syndrome, add Xuehai (SP 10) and Shuiquan (KI 5); for cases with Yin Deficiency syndrome, add Neiguan (PC 6) and Taixi (KI 3); for cases with Qi Deficiency syndrome, add Pishu (BL 20) and Zusanli (ST 36); and for cases with collapse syndrome, add Baihui (DU 20) and Qihai (RN 6).

Manipulation: Puncture with filiform needles by adopting reducing method in excessive Heat syndrome, and reinforcing method as well as moxibustion in Deficiency-Cold syndrome.

(3) Other therapy:

Scalp acupuncture: Select Lateral Line 3 of the forehead (MS 4) of the bilateral sides to be treated by twisting the needles simultaneously for a period of 3-5 minutes. Then, at an interval of 5 minutes, manipulate the needles twice in the same way as mentioned above. The treatment is performed once daily.

3. Abnormal fetal position

This indicates that fetus takes an incorrect position in the uterus after 30 pregnancy weeks. Prenatal examination often reveals abnormality of the fetal head and such abnormal fetal positions as breech presentation, transverse presentation or compound presentation. It is mostly seen in multipara or the pregnant women with an abdominal muscular relaxation. In TCM, it is called "incorrect fetal position".

Therapeutic method:

Prescription: Zhiyin (BL 67).

Manipulation: To be treated by applying moxibustion with moxa roll for 20 minutes, once or twice daily.

4. Infantile enuresis

Infantile enuresis indicates that involuntary discharge of urine still presents in the child reaching the age that the bladder can control the urination. In most cases, it refers to the enuresis that occurs once a week at least in children above 5 years old. Most children above 3 years old can control their urination. This disease is usually seen in girls and can be classified as two types: The primary and the secondary. The former is caused by deplayed maturity of the controlling effect of the bladder on discharging urine or functional small volume of the bladder; while the latter is usually caused by emotional injury, bladder diseases or systemic diseases, or by maldevelopment of the brain. In TCM, it is called "infantile enuresis" or "infantile nocturnal enuresis".

(1) Syndrome identification:

① Deficiency of the Kidney Yang syndrome: Enuresis during sleep which is noted after waking, accompanied with pale face, profuse, frequent and clear urine, or even cold limbs, aversion to cold, pale tongue, and a deep, slow and feeble pulse.

② Deficiency of both the Spleen Qi and the Lung Qi syndrome: Mostly occurring in patients just recovering from disease or those with a weak constitution, enuresis during sleep, frequent nocturnal urine with less volume, accompanied with pale and puffy face, listlessness, lassitude, poor appetite, loose stools, pale tongue and a soft or deep, fine pulse.

(2) Therapeutic methods:

① Deficiency of the Kidney Yang syndrome:

Prescription: Guanyuan (RN 4), Zhongji (RN 3), Shenshu (BL 23), Pangguangshu (BL 28), and Taixi (KI 3).

Manipulation: Puncture by using filiform needles with reinforcing method in combination with moxibustion.

② Deficiency of both the Spleen Qi and the Lung Qi syndrome:

Prescription: Qihai (RN 6), Taiyuan (LU 9), Zusanli (ST 36), and Sanyinjiao (SP 6).

Manipulation: Puncture by using filiform needles with reinforcing method in combination with moxibustion.

(3) Other therapies:

① Scalp acupuncture: Select Lateral Line 3 of forehead (MS 4), Lateral Line 1 of vertex (MS 8) and Lateral Line 2 of vertex (MS 9) to be needled subcutaneously. The needles are twisted for 1 minute and/or connected with the electric acupuncture instrument and then retained for 15 minutes.

② Auricular acupuncture: Select Kidney (EP-N4), Bladder (EP-N1), Subcortex (EP-E10) and Urethra (EP-N3) to be needled, 2-3 points each time with moderate stimulation, once daily. The needles are retained for 20 minutes.

5. Infantile diarrhea

Infantile diarrhea is a disease of the digestive tract with diarrhea as its main symptom. Its causes are various, and improper diet or infection of bacteria or viruses of the digestive tract can all lead to the disease. Mostly, it occurs in the young children below 2 years old and in the autumn, and is clinically characterized by increase of frequency of defecation, abdominal fullness, borborygmus, tart and foul stools or watery foamy stools mixed with indigested food and mucous fluid. In TCM, it is called "infantile diarrhea'.

(1) Syndrome identification:

① Damp-Heat syndrome: Loose, foul and yellow stools, abdominal pain, fever, thirst, burning sensation in anus, scanty and dark urine, yellow and greasy tongue coating, and a slippery, rapid pulse.

② Indigestion syndrome: Abdominal fullness and pain, diarrhea after the pain which is relieved by diarrhea, tart and foul stools like the rotten egg, eructation with a foul odour, vomiting the vomitus containing indigested food, dirty and greasy tongue coating, and a slippery and solid pulse.

③ Yang Deficiency syndrome: Recurrence and remission of diarrhea or protracted diarrhea with loose stools or indigested food, listlessness, lassitude, sallow complexion, or even cold limbs, incomplete closing of the eyes during sleep, pale tongue with whitish coating, and a fine and soft pulse.

(2) Therapeutic methods:

① Damp-Heat syndrome:

Prescription: Zhongwan (RN 12), Tianshu (ST 25), Zusanli (ST 36), Quchi (LI 11), and Neiting (ST 44).

Manipulation: Puncture by using filiform needles with reducing method.

② Indigestion syndrome:

Prescription: Zhongwan (RN 12), Jianli (RN 11), Tianshu (ST 25), Xuanji (RN 21), Qihai (RN 6), and Zusanli (ST 36).

Manipulation: Puncture by using filiform needles with reducing method.

186

③ Yang Deficiency syndrome:

Prescription: Pishu (BL 20), Shenshu (BL 23), Zusanli (ST 36), and Zhangmen (LR 13).

Manipulation: Puncture by using filiform needles with reinforcing method in combination with moxibustion with moxa roll.

(3) Other therapy:

Moxibustion: Select Guanyuan (RN 4), Tianshu (ST 25), Zhongwan (RN 12) to be treated by warming moxibustion while the child is in deep sleep. The moxibustion is applied to Zhongwan (RN 12) first for 20 minutes, then to Tianshu (ST 25) and Guanyuan (RN 4) for 30-50 minutes.

Diseases of the Ear, Eyes, Nose and Throat and Dermotological Diseases

1. Auditary vertigo

Auditary vertigo, also known as Menere's syndrome, is a disease marked by paroxysmal vertigo, undulant deafness, tinnitus, and a feeling of fullness in the ear, which is caused by labyrinthine hydrops. It is usually encountered in the young or middle aged people, and clinically, it is characterized by its sudden onset, a subjective feeling of spinning or rotating of the things around him or a feeling of spinning of himself, with a tendency to fall, which is aggravated by changes of position, accompanied with tinnitus, deafness, or nausea, vomiting and cold perspiration. In TCM, it is called "dizziness".

(1) Syndrome identification:

① Depletion of the Kidney essence syndrome: Frequent occurrence of vertigo, tinnitus, deafness, sharp ringing sound in the ear, more severe at night, soreness and weakness of the loins and knees, dream-disturbed sleep, emission, hectic fever, night sweat, poor memory, red tongue with little coating, and a fine, rapid or a wiry, fine pulse.

② Sinking of Qi due to Spleen Deficiency syndrome: Occurrence of vertigo at times, palpitation, shortness of breath, tinnitus, deafness, listlessness, disinclination to talk, sallow complexion, poor appetite, abdominal fullness, occasional loose stools, pale tongue with thin and whitish coating, and fine, soft and feeble pulse.

③ Liver Yang rising syndrome: Vertigo that is often induced by emotional upsets, vibration of the eyeballs, headache, distension of the ear, fullness in the chest and costal region, bitter taste in the mouth, dry throat, red face and eyes, or irritability, soreness and weakness of the loins and knees, feverish sensation over the palms and soles, insomnia, dream-disturbed sleep, red tongue with yellow coating, and a wiry, fine and rapid pulse.

④ Accumulation of Phlegm in the interior syndrome: Vertigo, heaviness of head as if being bound, blurred vision, chest distension, nausea or even vomiting thick fluid, lethargy, lassitude, pale tongue with white and greasy coating, and a soft or slippery pulse.

(2) Therapeutic methods:

① Depletion of the Kidney essence syndrome:

Prescription: Shenshu (BL 23), Taixi (KI 3), Ganshu (BL 18), Sanyinjiao (SP 6), Guanyuan (RN 4) and Xuanzhong (GB 39).

Manipulation: Puncture by using filiform needles with reducing method.

② Sinking of Qi due to Spleen Deficiency syndrome:

Prescription: Baihui (DU 20), Pishu (BL 20), Zusanli (ST 36), Zhongwan (RN 12), and Qihai (RN 6).

Manipulation: Puncture by using filiform needles with reinforcing method.

③ Liver Yang rising syndrome:

Prescription: Shenshu (BL 23), Taixi (KI 3), Taichong (LR 3), Xingjian (LR 2), Fengchi (GB 20), and Sanyinjiao (SP 6).

Manipulation: Puncture by using filiform needles with reinforcing method at Shenshu (BL 23), Taixi (KI 3) and Sanyinjiao (SP 6), and the reducing method at the rest points in this prescription.

④ Accumulation of Phlegm in the interior syndrome:

Prescription: Yinlingquan (SP 9), Zusanli (ST 36), Pishu (BL 20), Weishu (BL 21), Zhongwan (RN 12) and Fenglong (ST 40).

Manipulation: Puncture by using filiform needles with reducing method.

(3) Other therapy:

Auricular acupuncture: Select Xuanyundian (below Stomach, EP-M4), Kidney (EP-N4), Shenmen (EP-I1), Brain stem (EP-E1) and Occiput (EP-E5), to be needled and then twist the needle rapidly with strong stimulation, once daily. The needles are retained for 2- 3 hours.

2. Allergic rhinitis

Allergic rhinitis is an allergic disease involving the nasal mucous membrane, which is divided into two types: The seasonal and the non-seasonal. It is mainly seen in the young, and pollen, dust and stimuli of cold or hot wind serve as its main induction factors. Clinically, it is marked by sudden itching of nose, constant sneezing, profuse clear nasal discharge and such accompanying symptoms as headache and lacrimation. It often occurs paroxysmally, lasting from several minutes to years. In TCM, it is called "rhinitis".

(1) Therapeutic method:

Prescription: Shangyingxiang (EP-HN 8), Fengmen (BL 12), Hegu (LI 4) and Lieque (LU 7).

Manipulation: Puncture by twisting rapidly the needles with reducing method and strong stimulation, and uniform reinforcing and reducing method on the rest points in this prescription.

(2) Other therapies:

① Auricular acupuncture: Select Internal nose (EP-B6), Endocrine (EP-D1), Adrenal gland (EP-B8), Pinchuan (EP-E7), Lung (EP-O2) and Kidney (EP-N4), 3-4 points each time, once daily or once every other day. The needles are retained for 20 minutes.

② Moxibustion: Select Yintang (EX-HN 3), Shangxing (DU 13), Baihui (DU 20), Heliao (LI 19), Feishu (BL 17), Shenshu (BL 23), Zusanli (ST 36), 2-4 points each time, to be treated with suspending moxibustion with moxa roll for 20 minutes, once daily.

3. Pharyngitis

This is an inflammatory disease of the mucous membrane of the pharynx, its underlying tissues and the lymphatic tissues, which can be divided into the acute and the chronic. The acute pharyngitis is mostly the result of spread of the acute rhinitis downward to the pharynx, with acute onset, dryness, burning sensation and pain in the pharynx and such accompanying symptoms as fever, headache, poor appetite and aching of the limbs as its main clinical manifestations; while the chronic pharyngitis usually arises from repeated attack of the acute pharygitis, chronic inflammation of the adjacent tissues, frequent stimuli of chemical gas or dust and some chronic diseases, with various kinds of discomfort in the pharynx such as a feeling of foreign body obstructing in the throat, dryness, itching, mild burning sensation or pain in the pharynx. In TCM, it is called "throat obstruction".

(1) Syndrome identification:

① Attack of exogenous Wind-Heat syndrome: A feeling of foreign body obstructing in the throat, dryness, itching, burning pain in the pharynx, chills, fever, headache, red tongue with thin and yellow coating, and a floating and rapid pulse.

② Depletion of the Liver Yin and the Kidney Yin syndrome: Dryness and itching of pharynx which are mild in the morning and aggravated in the afternoon or at night, accompanied with feverish sensation over the palms and soles, hectic fever, night sweat, restlessness, insomnia, red tongue with little coating or without coating, and a fine and rapid pulse.

③ Exuberant Heat in the Lung and the Stomach syndrome: Severe swelling and pain in the pharynx, difficulty in swallowing, yellow, viscious and profuse sputum, accompanied with fever without aversion to cold, severe headache, dry mouth with desire for drinking, dark urine, constipation, red tongue with yellow thick coating, and a rapid and forceful pulse.

(2) Therapeutic methods:

① Attack of exogenous Wind-Heat syndrome:

Prescription: Shangyang (LI 1), Neiting (ST 44), Hegu (LI 4),

190

Lianquan (RN 23), and Tiantu (RN 22).

Manipulation: Puncture by using filiform needles with reducing method.

② Depletion of the Liver Yin and the Kidney Yin syndrome:

Prescription: Chize (LU 5), Yuji (LU 10), Taixi (KI 3), Zhaohai (KI 6), and Taichong (LR 3).

Manipulation: Puncture by adopting filiform needles with reinforcing method on Taixi (KI 3), Zhaohai (KI 6) and Taichong (LR 3), and the uniform reinforcing and reducing method on the rest points in this prescription.

③ Exuberant Heat in the Lung and the Stomach syndrome:

Prescription: Yuji (LU 10), Neiting (ST 44), Lianquan (RN 23).

Manipulation: Puncture by using filiform needles with reducing method.

(3) Other therapy:

Auricular acupuncture: Select Pharynx and larynx (EP-B4), Ear appex (EP-K12), Auricle 1-6 (EP-K1-6), Shenmen (EP-I1), Lung (EP-O2) and Kidney (EP-N4), 3-4 points each time, to be needled with moderate or strong stimulation, once daily. The needles are retained for 30 minutes.

4. Acute tonsilitis

Acute tonsilitis is a non-specific inflammation of the palatal tonsil, which is often accompanied with pharygitis of varying extents and degrees. It is mainly caused by hemolytic streptococcus B, and can be seen all the year round, although it is mainly seen in the spring and autumn. Clinically, this disease has a sudden onset, with chills, fever which may be 38℃-40℃, pain in the pharynx or during swallowing, redness and swelling of unilateral or bilateral tonsils covered with white pus spots, and such accompanying symptoms as headache, aching of the limbs, poor appetite and lassitude, as its manifestations. In TCM, it is called "A baby moth".

(1) Syndrome identification:

① Wind-Heat in the Lung channel syndrome: Pain in the pharynx with a dry and burning sensation, difficulty in swallowing, red and swollen tonsils, accompanied with fever, chills, headache, stuffy nose, red tongue tip and margin with yellowish coating, and a floating and rapid pulse.

② Exuberant Heat in the Lung and Stomach syndrome: Severe pain in the pharynx, which refers to the retroauricular region or the region below the jaw, red and swollen tonsils, which mainly involves the isthmus of fauces and covered with yellow or white pus spot, accompanied with high fever, severe thirst, cough with yellow and thick sputum, foul breathing, abdominal fullness, constipation, dark urine, red tongue with yellow and thick coating, and a full and rapid pulse.

(2) Therapeutic methods:

① Wind-Heat in the Lung channel syndrome:

Prescription: Tianrong (SI 17), Shaoshang (LI 1), Hegu (LI 4).

Manipulation: Puncture by using filiform needles with reducing method except for Shaoshang (LI 1) which is treated by pricking to cause bleeding.

② Exuberant Heat in the Lung and Stomach syndrome:

Prescription: Renying (ST 9), Yuji (LU 10), Hegu (LI 4), Neiting (ST 44), Quchi (LI 11), and Shangyang (LI 1).

Manipulation: Puncture by using filiform needles with reducing method except for Shangyang (LI 1) and Yuji (LU 10) which are pricked to cause bleeding.

(3) Other therapy:

Auricular acupuncture: Select Pharynx and larynx (EP-B4), Helix 4 (EP-K4), Helix 6 (EP-K6), and Tonsil 1-3 (EP-K7-9), to be needled with strong stimulation, once daily. The needles are retained for 30-60 minutes.

5. Chronic pharyngitis

Chronic pharyngitis is a chronic inflammation of the mucous membrane of the larynx caused by infection of common pathogens, which is classified as three types: The simple pharyngitis, the hypertrophic pharyngitis and the atrophic pharyngitis. It is usually caused by improper treatment of acute pharyngitis, repeated attack of the acute pharyngitis, over or improper use of the vocal fold, inhalation of poisonous gas or infection of the nose, pharynx or the mouth. Clinically, it is manifested as atonic and low voice, failure to talk long or even hoarseness, and is often accompanied with mild pain with a discomfort and dry feeling in the throat, cough with little sputum, etc. In TCM, it is called "chronic pharyngitis" and "hoarseness due to obstruction in the throat".

(1) Therapeutic method:

Prescription: Chize (LU 5), Taixi (KI 3), Lieque (LU 7), Zhaohai (KI 6), and Renying (ST 9).

Manipulation: Puncture by using filiform needles with reducing method on Taixi (KI 3) and Zhaohai (KI 6), and the uniform reinforcing and reducing method on the rest points in this prescription.

(2) Other therapy:

Moxibustion: Select Hegu (LI 4), Jiache (ST 6), Zusanli (ST 36), Feishu (BL 13), Fenglong (ST 40) and Zhaohai (KI 6) to be treated by suspending moxibustion with moxa roll for 5-10 minutes, 3-4 poinst each time, once daily or every other day.

6. Toothache

Toothache is one of the most commonly seen symptoms in mouth diseases, which is usually caused by dental caries, pulpitis or paradentoses. The pain is paroxysmal or dull in nature, severe at night, fixed or not fixed and is aggravated by exposure to cold or heat, intake of acid food or eating, and it is accompanied with thirst, headache, loose teeth, sore and foul odour in the mouth. In TCM, it is called "toothache".

(1) Syndrome identification:

① Wind-Fire syndrome: Toothache with swollen gum, aversion to cold, fever, thin and whitish coating, and a floating and rapid pulse.

② Excess Fire syndrome: Severe toothache, foul odour in the mouth, thirst, constipation, yellow and sticky coating, and a wiry pulse.

③ Deficiency-Fire syndrome: Dull toothache, which recurs frequently, loose teeth, no foul breath, red tongue tip, and a fine pulse.

193

(2) Therapeutic methods:

① Wind-Fire syndrome:

Prescription: Hegu (LI 4), Xiaguan (ST 7), Jiache (ST 6), Waiguan (Sj 5), Fengchi (GB 20).

Manipulation: Puncture by using filiform needles with reducing method.

② Excess Fire syndrome:

Prescription: Hegu (LI 4), Xiaguan (ST 7), Jiache (ST 6), Neiting (ST 44), Laogong (PC 8).

Manipulation: Puncture by using filiform needles with reducing method.

③ Deficiency-Fire syndrome:

Prescription: Hegu (LI 4), Xiaguan (ST 7), Jiache (ST 6), Taixi (KI 3), and Xingjian (LR 2).

Manipulation: Puncture by using filiform needle with reinforcing method on Taixi (KI 3), and the uniform reinforcing and reducing method on the rest points in this prescription.

(3) Other therapy:

Auricular acupuncture: Select Upper jaw (EP-A7), Lower jaw (EP-A5), Shenmen (EP-I1), Mouth (EP-M1) and Toothache (Ep-E2) to be treated with strong stimulation, with needles being retained for 20-30 minutes, or treated with needle-embedding.

7. Acute lymphangitis

Acute lymphangitis often results from invasion of the staphylococcus aureas or the hemolytic streptococcus into the lymph vessel through the lymph space from a wound in the skin or superficial mucous membrane or from a focus of infection. It is divided into two types: The reticular lymphangitis and the tubular lymphangitis, which are both manifested as redness, swelling, pain and hotness in the affected area, a red line spreading from the local lesion to the trunk of the body, accompanied with fever, chills, nausea and vomiting. In TCM, it is called "red line furuncle" or "red toxin".

(1) Therapeutic methods:

① Prescription: Shenzhu (DU 12), Lingtai (DU 10), Hegu (LI 4), Weizhong (BL 40), and Quchi (LI 11).

② Manipulation: Puncture by using filiform needle with reducing method, and prick at the interval of 1 cun from the starting point to the terminating point of the affected area along the red line to let out the affected blood.

(2) Other therapy:

Auricular acupuncture: Select Shenmen (EP-I1), Adrenal gland (EP-B8), Subcortex (EP-E10) and Occiput (EP-E5) to be needled with strong stimulation, once or twice a day. The needles are retained for 30 minutes.

8. Urticaria

Urticaria is a kind of commonly seen allergic disease of the skin, which arises from increase of the permeability and the dilation of the micrangium of the skin and the mucous membrane, and local edema due to exudation of the serum. It has something to do with the inheritary and the individual allergic prerequisite, and clinically, it is manifested as papura of varying sizes and numbers which emerge suddenly associated with severe sharp pain and itching. The papura may disappear in a period from several hours to 2 days, with temporal pigmentation remained, and it may occur in any part of the body. In TCM, it is called " hidden measles".

(1) Syndrome identification:

① Wind-Cold syndrome: Light red papura which becomes severe on exposure to wind or cold and can be relieved by warmth, severe in winter and mild in summer, thin and whitish tongue coating, and a floating, tense pulse.

② Wind-Heat syndrome: Red papura with a burning and severe itching sensation, which may coalesces into large patchy lesions or present streak after scraping, or more severe at night, with restlessness, insomnia, dry mouth, or accompanied with sore throat, red tongue with little coating, and a wiry, slippery and rapid pulse. In a protracted case, the papura is dark red in colour, mostly emerging in the regions of the wrist or waist where the watch or the belt are.

③ Wind-Dryness due to Blood Deficiency syndrome: Seen mostly in the aged or patients with a protractable disease. The papura is light red, fails to be cured for a long time, and is aggravated by physical strain. The tongue is pale with thin and little coating, and the pulse is wiry and fine.

④ Dampness obstructing in the Spleen and Stomach syndrome: Papura surrounded by edema, nausea, vomiting, abdominal pain and fullness, pale tongue with whitish coating, and a deep, fine and soft pulse.

⑤ Dysfunction of the Chong and Ren Channels syndrome: Papura that emerge 2-3 days before menstruation and disppear when the menstruation terminates, most in the lower abdomen, the lower back and the medial aspect of the thigh, accompanied with dark purplish tongue with thin and whitish coating, and a wiry and fine pulse.

(3) Therapeutic methods:

① Wind-Cold syndrome:

Prescription: Fengchi (GB 20), Quchi (LI 11), Fengmen (BL 12), and Xuehai (SP 10).

Manipulation: Puncture by using filiform needles with reducing method.

② Wind-Heat syndrome:

Prescription: Fengchi (GB 20), Dazhui (DU 14), Quchi (LI 11), Fengshi (GB 31), Fengmen (BL 12), and Xuehai (SP 10).

Manipulation: Puncture by using filiform needles with reducing method of strong stimulation.

③ Wind-Dryness due to Blood Deficiency syndrome:

Prescription: Hegu (LI 4), Quchi (LI 11), Tianshu (ST 25), Zusanli (ST 36), Sanyinjiao (SP 6), and Fengshi (GB 31).

Manipulation: Puncture by using filiform needles with uniform reinforcing and reducing method on Zusanli (ST 36) and Sanyinjiao (SP 6), and the reducing method with moderate or strong stimulation on the rest points.

④ Dampness obstructing in the Spleen and Stomach syndrome:

Prescription: Xuehai (SP 10), Geshu (BL 17), Pishu (BL 20), Sanyinjiao (SP 6), and Fengmen (BL 12).

Manipulation: Puncture by adopting filiform needles with reducing method on Fengmen (BL 12), and the reinforcing method on the rest points in this prescription.

⑤ Dysfunction of the Chong and Ren Channels syndrome:

Prescription: Guanyuan (RN 4), Geshu (BL 17), Xuehai (SP 10), Sanyinjiao (SP 6), Gongsun (SP 4), Qichong (ST 30) and Fengshi (GB 31).

Manipulation: Puncture by adopting filiform needles with reinforcing method on Guanyuan (RN 4) and Geshu (BL 17), and the reducing method on the rest points in this prescription.

(3) Other therapy:

Auricular acupuncture: Select Lung (EP-O2), Liver (EP-N9), Spleen (EP-N10), Shenmen (EP-I1), Adrenal gland (EP-B8) and Endocrine (EP-D1), 2-3 points each time, to be needled by using filiform needles with strong stimulation, once daily or once every other day. The needles are retained for 30 minutes.

9. Conjunctivitis

Conjunctivitis is a disease of the external eye marked by congestion, edema, dryness and discomfort, or formation of new vessels and follicles or papilla in the conjunctiva, which is mainly caused by bacterial infection or allergic reaction. Clinically, it is manifested as congestion and swelling of the conjunctiva, lacrimation, dryness, itching or other discomfort in the eyes, etc. In TCM, it is called epidemic red eye or "gold rebula".

(1) Syndrome identification:

① Affection of exogenous Wind-Heat syndrome: Reddness, swelling and pain of eyes, lacrimation, tearing, headache, fever, aversion to Wind, thin and yellowish tongue coating, and a floating and rapid pulse.

② Exuberant Fire in the Liver and Gallbladder syndrome: Redness, swelling and pain of eyes, lacrimation, lightphobia, bitter taste in the mouth, irritability, restlessness, constipation, red tongue tip or margin, and a wiry, rapid and forceful pulse.

(2) Therapeutic methods:

① Affection of exogenous Wind-Heat syndrome:

Prescription: Zanzhu (BL 2), Taiyang (EX-HN 5), Quchi (LI 11), and Hegu (LI 4).

Manipulation: Prick with three edged needle to cause bleeding on Taiyang (EX-HN 5), and puncture by using filiform needles with reducing method on the rest points in this prescription.

② Exuberant Fire in the Liver and Gallbladder syndrome:

Prescription: Tongziliao (GB 1), Taiyang (EX-HN 5), Hegu (LI 4), Xingjian (LR 2), and Xiaxi (GB 43).

Manipulation: Puncture with reducing method by using filiform needles.

(3) Other therapy:

Auricular acupuncture: Select Eye (EP-A 10), Liver (EP-N 9), Lung (EP-O2), Dachang (EP-M8), Taiyang (EP-E11) and Ear apex (EP-K12), 2-3 points each time, to be needled with moderate or strong stimulation, once daily. The needles are retained for 20 minutes.

10. Cataract

Cloudiness occurring in the lens of the eyeball by reason of aging, inheritary defect, immunological reaction, poisoning, metabolic disturbance or by reason of malnutrition in the affected part is known as cataract, which is divided into several different types, including the congenital cataract, senile cartaract, metabolic cataract, drug-induced cataract, traumatic cataract, complicated cataract, etc. At the initial stage, there is no subjective symptoms. Gradually, patient may have a subjective feeling of a fixed black spot floating or a mosquito flying in the front of his/her eye, or have a feeling of a layer of thin smoke or fog obstructing in the front of his/her eye. With the further development of the disease, the cloudiness of the lens becomes severe, and as a result, vision declines or even only light sense remains. In TCM, it is called "cataract with round rebulla".

(1) Syndrome identification:

① Deficiency of the Kidney and the Liver syndrome: Cloudiness of the eyeball, decline of vision, dizziness, tinnitus, soreness and weakness of the loins and knees, pale tongue, and a fine pulse.

② Deficiency of both Qi and Blood syndrome: Blurred vision, a few indistinct venules in the pupil, no strength to open or close the

198

eye, lassitude, indisclination to talk, dream-disturbed sleep with liability to waking, pale tongue, and a fine and feeble pulse.

③ Wind-Heat in the Liver Channel: Cloudiness of the eyeball due to traumatic injury or upward attack of Wind-Heat, bitter taste in the mouth, dry throat, distending pain of the eyes, headache, red tongue, and a wiry pulse.

(2) Therapeutic methods:

① Deficiency of the Kidney and the Liver syndrome:

Prescription: Dadun (LR 1), Taixi (KI 3), Sanyinjiao (SP 6), Mingmen (DU 4), Zanzhu (BL 2), and Jingming (BL 1).

Manipulation: Puncture by adopting filiform needles with uniform reinforcing and reducing method on Zanzhu (BL 2) and Jingming (BL 1), and the reinforcing method on the rest points in this prescription which can also be treated with moxibustion alternately in combination.

② Deficiency of both Qi and Blood syndrome:

Prescription: Baihui (DU 20), Xuehai (SP 10), Taibai (SP 3), Zusanli (ST 36), and Qiuhou (EX-HN 7),

Manipulation: Puncture by using filiform needls with reinforcing method except for Qiuhou (EX-HN 7) which can be treated by adopting both the acupuncture and moxbustion alternately.

③ Wind-Heat in the Liver Channel:

Prescription: Tongziliao (GB 1), Fengchi (GB 20), Guangming (GB 37), and Jingming (BL 1).

Manipulation: Puncture by using filiform needles with reducing method.

11. Central choroido-retinetis

Central choroido-retinitis is a disease marked by mild separation of the serous retina in maculae retina from the pigmented epithelium, which mostly affects one eye and the males of the young or middle aged. It has a tendency to recur, and clinically it is manifested as decline of vision, metamorphopsia, visual field defect, mild discoid serous retinal detechment in maxulae retina, with increase of the intensity of light reflection and disappearance of the light reflection in the depression of the center of the maculae retina. It is considered that it is related to disturbance of the venous circulation and increase of the permeability of the capillaries in the choroid. In TCM, it is called "blue blindness" or "vision confusion".

(1) Syndrome identification:

① Deficiency of both the Liver and the Kidney syndrome: Blurred vision, dark blue or grey spot in the front of eyes, dryness and discomfort of the eyes, pale tongue with little coating, and a deep and fine pulse.

② Deficiency of both Qi and Blood syndrome: Decline of vision, failure to see long, less brightness of the eyes, lassitude, feeble voice, indisclination to talk, pale tongue with whitish coating, and a fine and feeble pulse.

③ Accumulation of Dampness and Phlegm syndrome: Blurred vision, or metamorphopsia, chest stuffiness, heaviness of head, thick and greasy tongue coating, and a soft or slippery pulse.

(2) Therapeutic methods:

① Deficiency of both the Liver and the Kidney syndrome:

Prescription: Xingjian (LR 2), Taixi (KI 3), Baihui (DU 20), Jingming (BL 1), and Shenshu (BL 23).

Manipulation: Puncture by using filiform needles with uniform reinforcing and reducing method on Jingming (BL 1), and the reinforcing method on the rest points in this prescription.

② Deficiency of both Qi and Blood syndrome:

Prescription: Shangxing (DU 23), Xuehai (SP 10), Ganshu (BL 18), Jingming (BL 1), Qiuhou (EX-HN 7).

Manipulation: Puncture by using filiform needles with uniform reinforcing and reducing method on Jingming (BL 1) and Qiuhou (EX-HN 7), and the reinforcing method on the rest points which can also be treated by applying the acupuncture and moxibustion alternately.

③ Accumulation of Dampness and Phlegm syndrome:

Prescription: Fenglong (ST 40), Jiaxi (ST 41), Pishu (BL 20), Chengqi (ST 1), Shangxing (DU 23), and Zulinqi (GB 41).

Manipulation: Puncture by adopting filiform needles with reducing method on Chengqi (St 1) and Zulinqi (GB 41), and the uniform reinforcing and reducing method on the rest points in this prescription.

12. Myopia

This is an eye disease that patient can see the objects near clearly but fail to see the object at a distance distinctly, which is mainly caused by spasm of the cilliary muscle. It usually occurs in the adolescence and is related to the inheritary defect or improper use of the eyes after birth. Its clinical manifestations include decline of vision, failure to see things at a distance, headache, nausea, pain and distension of the eyeball, etc. In TCM, it is called "syndrome of failure to see far".

(1) Syndrome identification:

① Deficiency of both the Liver and the Kidney syndrome: Failure to see far, distending pain in the case of seeing a long time, dryness and discomfort in the eyes, dizziness, tinnitus, soreness and weakness of the loins and knees, reddish tongue with little coating, and a fine and deep pulse.

② Deficiency of both the Heart Yang and the Kidney Yang syndrome: Mostly caused by inheriditary defect, marked by failure to see far clearly, blurring of vision on seeing things near for a long time, accompanied with astigmatism, lustreless complexion, aversion to cold, cold limbs, pale tongue with whitish coating, and a deep and soft pulse.

(2) Therapeutic methods:

① Deficiency of both the Liver and the Kidney syndrome:

Prescription: Hegu (LI 4), Fengchi (GB 20), Guangming (GB 37), Ganshu (BL 18), Shenshu (BL 23), Jingming (BL 1), and Chengqi (ST 1).

Manipulation: Puncture by using filiform needles with uniform reinforcing and reducing method.

② Deficiency of both the Heart Yang and the Kidney Yang syndrome:

Prescription: Hegu (LI 4), Fengchi (GB 20), Guangming (GB 37), Xinshu (BL 15), Taixi (KI 3), Jingming (BL 1), and Chengqi (ST 1).

Manipulation: Puncture by using filiform needles with uniform reinforcing and reducing method except for patients with markable Yang Deficiency who should be treated with reinforcing method.

(3) Other therapy:

Auricular acupuncture: Select Eye (EP-A 10), Heart (EP-O 1), Liver (EP-N 9) and Kidney (EP-N 4) to be needled with moderate stimulation, once every other day. The needles are retained for 20 minutes.

Miscellaneous Diseases

1. AIDS

AIDS is a viral infectious disease caused by HIV (Human Immunodeficiency Virus), which is marked by progressive immunological deficiency. It has three transmission routes: Sexual contaction, infusion of blood products and diaplacental infection. It may affect the population of any age, but the young and the middle aged are most likely to be affected. Clinically, the manifestations of the disease may involve many sytems or organs, and have a tendency to become more and more severe. Repeated occurrence of fever, gradual loss of weight, lassitude, headache, unconsiousness, nausea, poor appetite, diarrhea, hemefecia, intractable cough, enlargement of the lymph nodes of the whole body, convulsion and dementia are the commonly seen symptoms of the disease. In TCM, there is no record about the disease in literature throughout ages, and it can be treated based on the treatment of such diseases as consumptive diseases or Blood disease in TCM.

(1) Syndrome identification:

① Attack of exogenous pathogen on the exterior syndrome: Fever, chills, general aching, cough, night sweat, lassitude, sore throat, poor appetite, thin and whitish tongue coating, and a floating and forceless pulse.

② Exuberance of toxic Heat syndrome: Persistent high fever, restlessness, thirst, lassitude, headache, red eyes, red, swollen and erosive skin, enlargement of lymph nodes, red tongue with yellow coating, and a rapid pulse.

③ Deficiency of both Qi and Yin syndrome: Listlessness, lassitude, shortness of breath, spontaneous sweating, feeble voice, dry cough with little sputum, feverish sensation over the palms, soles and chest, hectic fever, night sweat, pale face with red cheeks, reddish tongue with little coating, and a fine, feeble or a fine and rapid pulse.

④ Deficiency of both Qi and Blood syndrome: Feeble voice, spontaneous sweat, lassitude, pale or sallow complexion, dizziness, palpitation, pale tongue with whitish coating, and a fine and feeble pulse.

⑤ Stagnation of the Liver Qi syndrome: Emotional depression, irritability, chest distension, frequent sighing, being anxious, dry throat, pain in the costal region, emaciation, lassitude, dark red tongue with a thin and whitish coating.

⑥ Stagnation of Phlegm and Blood Stasis: Stabbing pain in the chest and costal region, abdominal masses or palpable masses in the hypochnodriac region which are aggravated by pressure, abdominal fullness, or even widely existed masses and nodules, scrofula, dull and dark face, dizziness, nausea, purplish and dark tongue dotted with ecchymosis, a whitish greasy coating, and a wiry, fine or a wiry slippery pulse.

⑦ Deficiency of both the Liver-Yin and the Kidney-Yin syndrome: Dizziness, vertigo, tinnitus, deafness, restlessness, irritability, soreness and weakness of the loins and knees, lassitude, hectic fever, night sweat, emaciation, red cheeks, dry mouth and throat, red tongue with little coating, and a fine, rapid pulse.

⑧ Deficiency of both the Spleen-Yang and the Kidney-Yang syndrome: Pale complexion, emaciation, lassitude, anorexia, diarrhea, soreness and weakness of the loins and knees, aversion to cold, cold limbs, impotence, emission, pale tongue with a white watery coating, and a feeble pulse.

⑨ Wind-Phlegm confusing the mind syndrome: Apathy, delayed reaction, or dementia, or sudden fall with unconsiousness, profuse sputum in the throat, convulsion, or deviation of eyes and mouth, hemiplegia, white, thick and greasy tongue coating, and a wiry slippery pulse.

⑩ Depletion of both Yin and Yang syndrome: Loss of weight, lustreless face, emaciation, dry mouth with little fluid, dizziness, tinnitus, or sticky perspiration, or pale complexion, cold limbs, spontaneous sweat or profuse cold sweating, feeble voice or even coma, light purple or red tongue with little coating, and a fine feeble or a feeble and indistinct pulse.

(2) Therapeutic methods:

① Attack of exogenous pathogen on the exterior syndrome:

Prescription: Lieque (LU 7), Hegu (LI 4), Fengchi (GB 20), Dazhui (DU 14), Zusanli (ST 36), and Guanyuan (RN 4).

Manipulation: Puncture by using filiform needles with reinforcing method on Zusanli (ST 36) and Guanyuan (RN 4), and reducing method on the rest points in this prescription.

② Exuberance of toxic Heat syndrome:

Prescription: Dazhui (DU 14), Quchi (LI 11), Zusanli (ST 36), Waiguan (SJ 5), and Hegu (LI 4).

Manipulation: Puncture by using filiform needles with reducing method.

③ Deficiency of both Qi and Yin syndrome:

Prescription: Zusanli (ST 36), Sanyinjiao (SP 6), Feishu (BL 13), Taiyuan (LU 9), and Gaohuangshu (BL 43).

Manipulation: Puncture by using filiform needles with reinforcing method.

④ Deficiency of both Qi and Blood syndrome:

Prescription: Guanyuan (RN 4), Zusanli (ST 36), Qihai (RN 6), Baihui (DU 20), Pishu (BL 20), and Xinshu (BL 15).

Manipulation: Puncture by using filiform needles with reinforcing method.

⑤ Stagnation of the Liver Qi syndrome:

Prescription: Qimen (LR 14), Taichong (LR 3), Ganshu (BL 18), Zhigou (SJ 6), and Zusanli (ST 36).

Manipulation: Puncture by using filiform needles with reducing method or uniform reinforcing and reducing method.

⑥ Stagnation of Phlegm and Blood Stasis:

Prescription: Dazhui (DU 20), Shaohai (HT 3), Qimen (LR 14), Shenshu (KI 23), and Zusanli (ST 36).

Manipulation: Puncture by adopting filiform needles with reducing method.

⑦ Deficiency of both the Liver-Yin and the Kidney-Yin syndrome:

Prescription: Zusanli (ST 36), Sanyinjiao (SP 6), Shenshu (BL 23), Taixi (KI 3), Mingmen (DU 4).

Manipulation: Puncture by using filiform needles with reinforcing method or uniform reinforcing and reducing method.

⑧ Deficiency of both the Spleen-Yang and the Kidney-Yang syndrome:

Prescription: Pishu (BL 20), Shenshu (BL 23), Mingmen (DU 4), Guanyuan (RN 4), and Zusanli (ST 36).

Manipulation: Puncture by using filiform needles with reinforcing method.

⑨ Wind-Phlegm confusing the mind syndrome:

Prescription: Shenmen (HT 7), Daling (PC 7), Yintang (EX-HN 3), and Fenglong (ST 40).

Manipulation: Puncture by using filiform needles with reinforcing method or uniform reinforcing and reducing method.

⑩ Depletion of both Yin and Yang syndrome:

Prescription: Shenshu (BL 23), Guanyuan (RN 4), Mingmen (DU 4), Taixi (KI 3), and Zusanli (St 36).

Manipulation: Puncture by using filiform needles with reinforcing method.

(3) Other therapy:

Moxibustion: Select Guanyuan (RN 4), Zusanli (ST 36), Feishu (BL 13), Pishu (BL 20), Shenshu (BL 23), Sanyinjiao (SP 6), Dazhui (DU 14), Bailao (EX-HN 15) and Mingmen (DU 4), 3-5 points each time, to be treated with 3 moxa rolls on each point, once every other day.

2. Addiction in smoking

Smoking of cigarette endangers the health of human body severely and may cause many kinds of disease. Years of clinical practice have shown that addiction in smoking can be treated effectively with acupuncture-moxibustion, which work through two ways: Inhibiting the addiction so that smokers lose their desire for smoking, and getting rid of the obstinence symptoms after giving up smoking such as restlessness, failure to concentrate one's mind, headache, lethargy, gastrointestinal discomfort and anxiety.

(1) Therapeutic methods:

① Prescription: Jieyanxue which is located at the midpoint between Yangxi (LI 5) and Lieque (LU 7).

② Manipulation: Puncture by adopting filiform needle 0.3 cun perpendicularly with strong stimulation, once daily with the needle retained for 30 minutes.

(2) Other therapies:

① Auricular acupuncture: Select Mouth (EP-M1), Shenmen (EP-I1) and Lung (EP-O2) to be needled with moderate stimulation, 3 times a week with the needle retained for 15 minutes in each treatment. Needling-embedding is applicable.

② Electric acupuncture: Select Hegu (LI 4) and Zusanli (ST 36) to be needled. After the feeling of gaining Qi is obtained, connect the needles with the electric acupuncture instrument and then exert the current with continuous waves at an intensity that patient can bear, once daily with the needle retained for 20 minutes.

Acupuncture Anaesthesia

*A*cupuncture anaesthesia is a new non-drug method to induce anaesthesia. It works by inducing the human body to produce a series of adaptive, holistic and ordered regulatory processes by which to change the original functional state of the human body, enhance the threshold of tolerance to pain, increase the adaptive and regulatory capacities of the important life systems including the nervous system, circulatory system, the digestive system and the immunological system so that patient can accept surgical operation safely in a conscious state.

A Survery of Acupuncture Anaesthesia

1. Actions and characteristics

Through years of clinical observation and study of its mechanism in China, five kinds of actions of acupuncture in inducing anaesthesia have been confirmed: ① analgesic effect, ② counteracting the pulling reaction of viscus, ③ counteracting traumatic shock, ④ counteracting operative infection, and ⑤ promoting recovery of the traumatic tissues after operation.

Meanwhile, the acupuncture anaesthesia have five major characteristics: ① patient is kept awake during operation, still having various kinds of basically normal sensory or motor functions excepts dysethenia, so he/she can coordinate well with surgeons to ensure the normal performance of the operation; ② it is a safety anaesthesic method. According to incomplete statistics, more than two millions cases have been operated with acupuncture anaesthesia in China, and unexpected death by reason of acupuncture anaesthesia have not been reported jet; ③ acupuncture anaesthesia has a positive action of counteracting the unfavorable conditions occurring in operation through increasing the adaptive and regulatory functions of the circulatory system, the digestive system and the immunological system, so it has the effect of counteracting the traumatic shock and operative infection as well as improving postoperative inhibition of the patient; ④ it brings about no side or toxic effect, and has a wide indications; and ⑤ its anesthesic effect has a certain physiological limitation and varies with individuals, which may cause incomplete anaesthesia, inadequate relaxation of muscles or pulling reaction of the viscus. Besides, it is difficult to predict the anaesthesic effect of acupuncture, and this may bring about some troubles to the operation or the anesthetist.

2. Method of acupuncture anaesthesia

(1) Preoperative preparation: Before operation, medical staffs should determine an ascertained schedule for the acupuncture anaesthesia, estimate various conditions that possibly occur and determine the appropriate corresponding measures to be adopted. As patient is of consciousness during operation, the characteristics, method, procedures, effect of the acupuncture anaesthesia as well as the discomfort that may happen to the patient should be explained to the patient, so that he/she is mentally prepared and know how to coordinate with doctors in the operation such as he/she knows to breathe in deeply while his/her chest is being opened. In addition, a trial acupuncture should be performed before operation in order to know the situation of gaining Qi and the tolerant ability of the patients to

the acupuncture to guarantee that proper stimulating method as well as appropriate stimulation is employed.

(2) Principle to select points: Selecting the points that produces the feeling of gaining Qi quickly or produces severe sourness and distension but produces no pain or bleeding and asking patient to take a proper position which doesn't exert any unfavorable influence on the doctor's operation form the basic principles to select points. The points of the fourteen channels should be selected for body acupuncture, which can be carried out in three different ways.

① Selection of points along the distribution route of channels, which means to select the acupoints and channels closely related to the cutting position and the viscera to be operated, in accordance with the theroy that disease along the distributing route of a channel can be treated by using the points of the channel. For example, Hegu (LI 4) of the hand Yangming channel can be selected in inducing anaesthesia in tooth extraction.

② Selection of the local area, which means that the acupoints adjacent to the region to be operated can be selected.

③ selection of points in the light of nerve theory, which means to select the acupoints distributed over or adjacent to the dominated area of the same neural segment or to select the points according to the distribution of the nerve trunk, or to stimulate the nerve trunk directly. For example, Futu (LI 18) and Neiguan (PC 6) can be selected to induce anaesthesia in operation of the thyroid gland, which is an example of selecting the points according to the neural segment, and Jiquan (HT 1) can be selected in operation of the upper limbs which is an example of selecting the acupoints that are located at the nerve trunks. The above-mentioned three methods may be adopted along or jointly.

There are also three methods to select acupoints in auricular acupuncture anaesthesia. The first one is that the points can be selected in accordance with theory of Zang-Fu organs. For example, Lung (EP-O2) may be adopted in cutting skin and sewing skin. The second is that the points may be selected in the light of the operation locale. For example, Appendix (EP-M7) may be selected in appendectomy. And, the third is that the points may be selected in accordance with inervation and anatomical physiology. For example, Mouth (EP-M1) and Ermigen point may be selected in the operation on the viscus in the abdominal cavity because the viscus are dominated by the vegetative nerve. These three methods mentioned-above may also be adopted alone or jointly.

Mostly, the points of the affected side are adopted in body acpuncture or auricular acupuncture anaesthesia, although the points of the bilateral sides may be employed sometimes.

(3) Stimulation methods:

① Application of needling manipulations: The needles should be manipulated evenly and steadily. Usually, twisting-rotating manipulation or combined twisting-rotating manipulation and lifting-inserting manipulation are adopted in body acupuncture; while the needles can only be twisted and rotated in auricular acupuncture. The manipulation frequency should be 120-200 times per minutes, at an agle between 90°-360°, and the amplitude of the lifting and inserting should be between 5 mm and 10 mm. It is required that the patients must be kept in a state of gaining Qi.

② Electric acupuncture anaesthesia: It is manipulated in the same way as the electric acupuncture applied in treatment of disease. Usually, intense waves are applied with a stimulation that patient can bear.

In addition, the anaesthsia may also be induced by hydro-acupuncture, point-finger-pressing, instrument-pressing and electrode anaesthesia, which may take the place of the acupuncture anaesthesia.

③ Induction and needle-retaining: Stimulation on the acupoints selected for some time in advance of the operation is known induction, which may last from 20 to 30 minutes. The induction may be divided into general induction and the induction with the emphasis placed on several points. The former indicates that all the acupoints selected are needled in accordance with their sequence in a relatively longer time; while the latter indicates that manipulations of needles are perform on some key acupoints, which should be done 5 minutes before the operation. Usually light stimulation should be conducted during operation, but the stimulation may be strengthened at the acupoints which are sensitive, and in some operation which may bring about mild stimulation to the patient, manipulation or connection of the needles with the electric acupuncture instrument may be stopped temporarily. For example, the needles may be retained without any manipulations during the cerebral operation when the meninges is insected.

3. Supplementary administration of drugs

Administration of drugs before operation may not be necessary in a small operation with acupuncture anaesthesia or anordinary operation on which acupuncture anaesthesia has a stable effect. However, drugs should be applied in big operations in accordance with the patient's tolerance to the acupuncture, the patient's constitutions and mental states, so as to relax the emotional stress that happens to the patient during operation and enhance the effect of the acupuncture anaesthesia. As one of the anaesthesic method, acupuncture anaesthesia still has the shortcoming of causing incomplete anaesthesia, so it is very important to administrate drugs appropriately for both the development of acupuncture anaesthesia and the entire interests of patient. The commonly used drugs in advance of operation include analgesics for the central nervous system of which luminal sodium, usually administered by intramuscular injection one hour before the operation, is the mostly frequently adopted; the neuroleptics, of which diazepam, pethidine, etc. , applied by muscular injection, intravenous drip ot intravenous injection, are the most frequently adopted. Drugs that are applied during operation may be the sedatives, anelgesics, or muscle relaxants, depending on patient's response and the concrete situations of the operation. The drugs applied during operation must be given in due time, or before violent response happens to patients, so that a satisfactory effect can be obtained. The dosages of the drugs, especially those of the muscles relaxant, must be strictly limited.

4. Indications

Since the acupuncture anaesthesia came into being in 1958, it has been adopted to induce anaesthesia early or later in almost all kinds of surgical operations, including the operations on the head, the five sensory organs, the face, the neck, the chest, the abdomen and the four limbs. In its clinical application, the acupuncture anaesthesia has been carefully studied in more than 100 kinds of operations of different clinical branches in China. Of the 100 or more surgical operations, acupuncture anaesthesia is frequently adopted in about 20-30 kinds of operations with a stable anelgesic effect and a success rate of 80%-90%. According to the statistics of more than ten thousands cases made by the All-China Cooperative Group of the Study of Head, Galucoma, Thyroid Gland, Lung, Stomach and Uterus, the surgical operations can be divided into three kinds in accordance with the anaesthesic effect of acupuncture: ① Acupuncture anaesthesia has a stable anelgesic effect on the surgical operation of the thyroid gland, operation of the anterior cranial depression, cesarean section, tooth extraction, partial gastrectomy in a state of anaesthesia with both the Laser and the acupuncture anaesthesia, ligation of oviduct, and pneumonectomy. So, acupuncture anaesthesia should be widely spread in these operations; ② The acupuncture anaesthesia can be used as an anaesthesic method but its effect is not stable in such operations as maxillary sinus radical treatment, appendectomy, hysterectomy, and subtotal gastrectomy; and ③ Acupuncture anaesthesia is not so effective for orthopedic operations on the four limbs, operations on the perineum, etc. It is generally believed that acupuncture has a better anelgesic effect on and is indicated for the operations of the head, face, neck and chest with a broad indication, the operation of the diseases with a definite diagnosis and simple locale during which entensive exploration is not necessary or the muscles relaxation is not so strictly stressed, the operation in patients who are not indicated for drug anaesthesia or are allergic to the drugs, or the operations in patients who produce a strong feeling of gaining Qi and have a higher tolerance to pain or whose threshold of pain is enhanced in the acunpunture induction performed before the operation.

Acupuncture Anaesthesia Adopted
In Commonly Adopted Operations

1. Operation of the thyroid gland

(1) Prescription: Hegu (LI 4), Neiguan (PC 6), and Futu (LI 18).

(2) Manipulation: All the above points are manipulated through electric acupuncture instrument. The bilateral Hegu (LI 4) and Neiguan (PC 6) are used and manipulated with a frequency of 2-8 HZ, while the bilateral Futu (LI 18) are adopted and manipulated with a frequency of 40-80 HZ. The induction should last 15-30 minutes.

(3) Attentions:

① Acupuncture anaesthesia should be adopted with great care in the operation on the huge thyroid enlargement, which is often accompanied with symptoms of obstruction of the respiratory tract and malacia and detelectasis of the trachea.

② Such drugs as luminal sodium can be administered as a supplement in advance of operation in accordance with the patients' condition, and local anaesthesics should be applied in the case of pain being felt when an injection needle is inserted into the skin of the cutting edge while the skin is incised.

2. Radical treatment of the thyroid cancer

(1) Prescription: Hegu (LI 4), Neiguan (PC 6), Yifeng (SJ 7), and Xiaguan (ST 7).

(2) Manipulation: All the above points are stimulated by using an electric acupuncture instrument with a frequency of 4-8 HZ, and the induction should last 30 minutes.

(3) Attentions: The attentions are the same as those for the opertion of the thyroid enlargement.

3. Operation of the cervical vertebrae

(1) Prescription: Futu (LI 18), Waiguan (SJ 5), and Hegu (LI

4).

(2) Manipulation: The above points are to be stimulated by the constant waves of the electric impulse produced by an acupuncture anaesthesia equipment, at a frequency of 2-3 HZ on Hegu (LI 4) and Waiguan (TE 5) and a frequency of 100 HZ on Futu (LI 18). The induction should last 20-30 minutes.

(3) Attentions:

① Keeping the reaspiratory tract smooth: The respiration should be observed by means of proper equipments. In the case of respiratory inhibition, pressor oxygen inhalation should be given; in the case of profuse ozzing of blood, blood transfusion should be administered to maintain the stability of circulation; in the case of sudden decrease of blood pressure, hemopiesics must be given in time to keep the blood pressure in a normal state; and in such operations as decompression of the vertebral lamina and plastic operation of the vertebral lamina, dexamethasone sodium phosphate 20 mg may be given by intravenous drip to prevent edema of spinal cord.

② Administering drugs in advance of operation: Before the operation, scopolamine should be given in the light of the patient's condition, and before the skin is to be cut, pethidine at a dose of 1 mg/kg of body weight, or fentanyl at a dose 0.1 mg/kg of body weight, may be given by intravenous drip. In the case of emotional stress or with cardiovascular diseases, luminal sodium or diazepam should be given by intravascular injection. The cutting edge in this operation is usually big and tends to produce profuse hemorrhage, so, 1.23%-1.25% procaine with several drops of adrenalin added can be applied to the cutting edge.

4. Operation of the anterior cranial depression

(1) Prescription: Quanliao (SI 18), Jinmen (BL 63) and Taichong (LR 3).

(2) Manipulation: All the above acupoints are manipulated with electric acupuncture instrument. Quanliao (LI 18) is stimulated at a frequency of 8-16 HZ by connecting with the cathod while the anode is connected with the ear lobe. Insert a 2 cun long needle 1 cun perpendicularly at the point directly below the outer canthus and at the

214

level of the ala nasi, then adjust the depth of the needle tip to be the muscular layer and insert 2 cm obliquely toward the outer canthus along the surface of the zygomatic bone. Jinmen (BL 63) is connected with the cathod and Taichong (LR 3) with the anode to be stimulated at a frequency of 2-4 HZ.

(3) Attentions:

① Administration of supplementary drugs: Give luminal sodium 0.1 g by intramuscular injection before operation; give luminal sodium as well as diazepam in cases with a history of epilepsy episode, pethidine by intramuscular injection or intravenous drip at a dose of 1 mg/kg; give injection on Neiguan (PC 6) with maxolon in cases with nausea and vomiting during operation.

② The electric stimulation produced by the acupuncture electric instrument should be within the limit that patient can tolerate. The needles may be retained with the electric stimulation ceased after the dura mater of the spinal cord is incised, and the stimulation should be resumed again when the dura mater is to be sewed.

③ Injury to the dura mater must be avoided when the bone flat is folded, and the bone flat should be prevented from being separated from the muscle bluntly. The operation field should be washed with warm saline solution. Cutaneous, muscular or dura mater bleeding should be stopped with a hemostatic clamp instead of a monopolar coagulation forceps.

5. Tooth extraction

(1) Prescription: Xiaguan (ST 7), Jiache (ST 6), Quanliao (SI 18), Hegu (LI 4).

(2) Manipulation: The needles are stimulated with electric impulse of constant double-direction sharp waves or square waves at a frequency of 200 HZ. The intensity should be that patient can bear or that no muscular spasm occurs. The induction should last 1-10 minutes.

(3) Attentions: Faint during tooth extraction should be avoided. The operation must be carried out stably, precisely, gently and quickly.

6. Pneumonectomy

(1) Prescription: Sanyangluo (SJ 8) to Ximen (PC4), Xiayifeng, Ren Channel and Du Channel.

(2) Points jointly used: Add Houxi (SI 3), Zhigou (SJ 6), Shugu (BL 65), Zulinqi (GB 41) and Neiguan (PC 6) when the skin is to be cut; add Zhigou (SJ 6), Neiguan (PC 6), and Taichong (LR 3) when the periost is to be peeled; add Hegu (LI 4), Zhigou (SJ 6) and Zulinqi (GB 41) when the drainage-tube is to be installed; add Ximen (PC 4), Houxi (SI 3), Neiguan (PC 6) and Taichong (LR 3) in the case of dyspnea when the thoracic cavity is opened; and add Juji (LU 10) and Taibai (SP 3) when cough occurs following opening of the thoracic cavity.

(3) Manipulation: Puncture 1-2 cun perpendicularly on Xiayifeng and 3-4 cun subcutaneously on the Ren and Du Channels first; then stimulate the points electrically in a routine way by connecting the Sanyangluo (SJ 8) with the annode and Xiayifeng with the cathode at a low frequency, and by connecting Ren Channal with the annode and the Du Channel with the cathode at a high frequency. The above jointly used points are treated with reducing method through twisting the needles by hand. The electric frequency usually ranges from 200-2000 HZ, which is adopted differently in accordance with the different procedures of the operation.

(4) Attentions:

① Acupuncture anaesthesia in pneumonectomy has some indications. It is not suggested in patients with cardiovascular diseases, hypertension that fails to be controlled, diabetes, and severe damage of the function of the heart and the lung, or in those with abnormal mental states.

② Administer drugs as a supplement. Give luminal sodium 0.1 g and atropine 0.4 mg by subcutaneous injection or intramuscular injection 1 hour before the operation and pethidine 50-75 mg by intravenous drip 10 minutes before the operation; immerse the subcutaneous tissues with saline containing a small amount of adrenalin when the skin is to be cut; block the transmission of the intercostal nerve with 1% of procaine when the periost is to be peeled; and give a small dose of lidocaine to block hilus of lung when it is handled.

216

During the operation, half dose of pethidine may be added.

③ Patient should do more breathing exercise before operation in order to increase the vital capacity and the maximal ventilatory volume. While the thoracic cavity is opened or closed, doctors must be very careful with gentle manipulations. Sideration, electric knife, blunt separation and strong pulling must be avoided. And during the operation, the respiratory tract must be kept unobstructed.

7. Resection of the esophageal carcinoma

(1) Prescription: Sanyangluo (SJ 8), Xiayifeng, the Ren Channel and the Du Channel.

(2) Manipulation: The above acupoints or channels are to be stimulated by electric acupuncture with Xiayifeng and Sanyangluo (SJ 8) as one group and the Ren Channel and the Du Channel as other group. The former group is treated by adopting the low frequency; while the latter is treated by adopting the high frequency. See the "Manipulations" for pneumonectomy for concrete manipulations of the above acupoints.

(3) Attentions:

① The states of the patient's circulatory system, the respiratory system and the general conditions must be examined carefully. If necessary, proper treatments should be given before the operation. And, during the operation, the patient's condition must be kept under strict observation, and proper measures must be prepared.

② Usually carcinoma in the upper or middle portion of the esophagus is not suggested to be operated with acupuncture anaesthesia. If the acupuncture anaesthesia is employed, tracheal cannula should be adopted simultaneously in order to maintain the normal respiration.

8. Partial gastrectomy

(1) Prescription: Zusanli (ST 36), Shangjuxu (ST 37), needlings beside the cutting edge.

(2) Manipulation: The above points are to be stimulated with electric acupuncture at a frequency of 5-20 HZ on Zusanli (ST 36) and Shangjuxu (ST 37). The needles beside the cutting edge are inserted subcutaneously from the upper part to the lower part. The

needles may be inserted along the costal margins of the right and the left or beside the straight muscle of the abdomen and then connect with the cathod and the annode respectively to be stimulated at a frequency of 20-100 HZ. The induction should last 30 minutes.

(3) Attentions:

① Administer drugs as supplement. Drugs applied before operation include luminal sodium 0. 1 g and atropine 0. 5 mg which are given by intramuscular injection 30 minutes before cutting the skin, pethidine at a dose 1-1. 5 mg/kg body weight which is given by intravenous drip 10 minutes before cutting skin. Drugs applied during operation include 0. 5% procaine, 1-3 ml, which is infused to the local area in such key procedures of the operation as cutting or sewing the peritoneum, ligating the left or the right gastric artery, dissecting the peripheral mucosa of the ulcerous tissues, freeing the duodenum or closing the abdomnial cavity with muscle tone. Be sure to keep the patient's respiration under strict observation.

② The stimulation arising from the peritoneum or ligation of the right and left gastric artery is of great significance for the success or not of the operation. laparotomical instrument as well as intra-abdominal exploration are not suggested unless they are necessary.

③ Acupuncture anaesthesia is suitable for patients with bleeding of the upper digestive tract or duodenal obstruction caused by gastric ulcer, especially the aged patients with general weakness or shock. But it is not applicable to those with an unstable emotional state, complicated disease or requiring to be explored extensively during the operation.

9. Laparotomy ventrotomy

(1) Prescription: Sanyinjiao (SP 6), Waimadian (on the lateral aspect of the lower leg, one finger breadth from the anterior crest of the tibia, at the midpoint of the line connecting the head of the fibula and the prominence of the external malleolus), and needlings beside the cutting edge.

(2) Manipulation: Puncture perpendicularly 1-1. 5 cun on Sanyinjiao (SP 6) and 0. 5-1 cun on Waimadian, and subcutaneously 2-3 cun beside the cutting edge. The frequency of the electric impulse

218

adopted is 2 HZ in Sanyinjiao (SP 6) and Waimadian, and 800 HZ beside the cutting edge. The induction should last 15-30 minutes.

(3) Attentions:

① Ask patient to exacuate her bladder; doctor should know the position of the fetal head, and uterus contraction agent should be injected through the wall of uterus when the largest part of the fetal head is being delivered.

② Give luminal sodium 0.1 mg and atropine 0.25 mg by intramuscular injection before operation. Immerse the local area with 0.5% of procaine and then give pethidine at a dose of 1 mg/kg of body weight by intravenous drip when the skin is to be cut. 1% tetracaine, 1-2ml, should be sprayed or smeared with a cotton ball in the case of peritoneum and viscus dragging pain.

10. Ligation of oviduct

(1) Prescription: Brain of the ear points and Lung (EP-O2), Shenmen (EP-I1) and Uterus (EP-I5), and needlings beside the cutting edge.

(2) Manipulations: Employ the electric anaesthesia to stimulate with constant waves at a frequency of 25-50 HZ on the ear points and 100 HZ on needlings beside the cutting edge. The needles should be retained with the electricity stopped when the ovidust is to be picked up from the abdo ri..al cavity and ligated.

(3) Attentions:

① Have a knowledge of the patient's condition and her disease history, perform the gynecological and the ordinary examinations, and determine the operation schedule.

② See the application of drugs as a supplement for the laparotomy ventrotomy.

针灸疗法

编　　著　张登部
　　　　　杜广中
译　　者　路玉滨
　　　　　卢兖伟
责任编辑　李　宇

＊

山东科学技术出版社出版
济南市玉函路 16 号　邮政编码　250002
山东滨州新华印刷厂印刷
中国国际图书贸易总公司发行
中国北京车公庄西路 35 号
北京邮政信箱第 399 号　邮政编码　100044

＊

1996 年(大 32 开)　1 版 1 次
ISBN 7－5331－1851－0
R・539
07200
14－E－3020P